Exercise and Cardiac Death

Medicine and Sport

Vol. 5

Editor: E. JOKL, Lexington, KY
Assistant Editor: M. HEBBELINCK, Brussels

Published for and on behalf of the Research Committee, International Council of Sport and Physical Education, UNESCO

University Park Press · Baltimore · London · Tokyo

Exercise and Cardiac Death

Editors: E. Jokl and J.T. McClellan

With 37 figures and 8 tables

University Park Press · Baltimore · London · Tokyo   1971

Originally published by S. Karger AG, Basel, Switzerland
Distributed exclusively in the United States of America and Canada by
University Park Press, Baltimore, Maryland

Library of Congress Catalog Card Number 78–149556
Standard Book Number 0-8391-0529-0

Medicine and Sport

Previous Volumes

Vol. 1 Exercise and Altitude
Edited by E. JOKL and P. JOKL, Lexington, Ky. VIII + 200 p., 47 fig., 24 tab., 1968.
Vol. 2 Biomechanics
Technique of Drawings of Movement and Movement Analysis.
First International Seminar of Biomechanics, Zurich 1967
Edited by J. WARTENWEILER, Zurich; E. JOKL, Lexington, Ky. and M. HEBBELINCK,
Brussels, XXIV + 352 p., 216 fig., 17 tab., 1968.
Vol. 3 Biochemistry of Exercise
First International Symposium on Exercise Biochemistry, Brussels 1968
Edited by J. R. POORTMANS, Brussels, X + 384 p., 127 fig., 83 tab., 1969.
Vol. 4 Physical Activity and Aging
With special reference to the effect of exercise and training on the natural history
of arteriosclerotic heart disease
Edited by D. BRUNNER, Tel Aviv-Jaffa and E. JOKL, Lexington, Ky.
XII + 315 p., 98 fig., 71 tab., 1970.

S. Karger · Basel · München · Paris · London · New York · Sydney
Arnold-Böcklin-Strasse 25, CH-4000 Basel 11 (Switzerland)

© Copyright 1971 by S. Karger AG, Verlag für Medizin und Naturwissenschaften, Basel
Printed in Switzerland by Imprimeries Réunies S.A., Lausanne
Blocks: Steiner & Co., Basel
Binding by Max Grollimund, Basel

Table of Contents

Introduction.   VI

JOKL, E. and MCCLELLAN, T. J.: Asymptomatic Cardiac Disease Causing
Sudden Death in Association with Physical Activity (I)   1

JOKL, E. and MELZER, L.: Acute Fatal Non-Traumatic Collapse During Work
and Sport (II).   5

JOKL, E. and SUZMAN, M. M.: Mechanisms Involved in Acute Fatal Non-
traumatic Collapse Associated with Physical Exertion (III)   19

JOKL, E. and MCCLELLAN, J. T.: Sudden Cardiac Death of Pilots in Flight (IV)   25

JOKL, E. and GREENSTEIN, J.: Fatal Coronary Sclerosis in a Boy of Ten
Years (V)   64

JOKL, E. and MELZER, L.: Rheumatic Fever Following Athletic Trauma (VI)   67

GLANCY, D. L.; YARNELL, PH. and ROBERTS, W. C.: Traumatic Left Ventricular
Aneurysm (VII)   71

JOKL, E. and NEWMAN, B.: Death of a Wrestler (VIII)   81

MCCLELLAN, J. T. and JOKL, E.: Congenital Anomalies of Coronary Arteries
as Cause of Sudden Death Associated with Physical Exertion (IX) . . .   91

JOKL, E.: Sudden Death After Exercise Due to Myocarditis (X)   99

JAMES, T. N.; FROGGATT, P. and MARSHALL, T. K.: Sudden Death in Young
Athletes (XI)   102

PUGH, L. G. C. E.: Deaths from Exposure on Four Inns Walking Competition,
March 14–15, 1964 (XII).   112

SCHRIER, R. W.; HENDERSON, H. S.; TISHER, C. C. and TANNEN, R. L.: Nephropathy Associated with Heat Stress and Exercise (XIII)   121

JOKL, E.: Sudden Death During Exercise Due to Congenital Anomaly of Aortic Valve (XIV) 148

JOKL, E. and MACKINTOSH, R. H.: Sudden Death of Young Athlete from Rupture of Ascending Aorta (XV) 150

JOKL, E. and CLUVER, E. H.: Sudden Death of a Rugby International after a Test Game (XVI) 153

GIKNIS, F. L.; HOLT, D. E.; WHITEMAN, H. W.; SINGH, M. D.; BENCHIMOL, A. and DIMOND, E. G.: Myocardial Infarction in Twenty-Year-Old Identical Twins (XVII) 159

GREEN, J. R.; KROVETZ, L. J.; SHANKLIN, D. R.; DEVITO, J. J. and TAYLOR, W. J.: Sudden Unexpected Death in Three Generations (XVIII) 166

Introduction

The clarification of the problem of sudden cardiac death associated with physical exertion represents the most important single contribution made by clinical sportsmedicine to internal medicine so far. It is now possible to differentiate between the natural history of heart disease in patients who during their illness seek medical advice, as contrasted to that of persons in whom the terminal collapse represents the first manifestation of the cardiac affliction. The evidence presented in this volume relates to the latter category and its clinical implications. It also draws attention to the fact that impairment of exercise capacity is not a reliable prognostic criterion in cardiology as shown by the description of cases in which death occurred following outstanding athletic performances. Furthermore, the data under review demonstrate that the discovery *post mortem* even of *gross pathological changes* in the heart does not necessarily suffice to explain the fatal seizures. *Supplementary factors* are invariably involved, such as intercurrent infections (e.g. those discussed in VI and X), trauma to the chest, e.g. those discussed in V, VII, and VIII, or thermic stress, e.g. those discussed in XII and XIII [4]. That the *timing* of cardiac seizures and their particular clinical characteristics do not occur fortuitously is shown by observations of simultaneously developing acute circulatory failure in identical twins and in several members of the same family, e.g. those discussed in XVI and XVII [3, 7].

The contents of the volume have been arranged as follows: The opening section entitled 'Asymptomatic Cardiac Diseases Causing Sudden Death in Association with Physical Activity' summarizes 4 pathological syndromes that have been discovered during autopsy in cases of sudden unexpected death associated with physical exertion, namely *coronary arterio-* and *athero-sclerosis*, mostly associated with myocardial changes; *congenital anomalies of the coronary arteries; myocarditis;* and *cardiac tumors.* In Section II we report on 64 autopsies conducted after fatal seizures of the kind under study. Invariably, morphological manifestations of diseases of the circulatory system were found. Section III is devoted to a discussion of *trigger mechanisms* presumably responsible for the onset of the terminal syncope.

By far the most frequent *post-mortem* findings in cases of sudden cardiac death associated with exercise is *coronary athero-* and *arterio-sclerosis.* In Sections IV, V, and VIII the problem is elaborated in connection with observations of sudden cardiac deaths of pilots in flight, of a case of sudden death of a boy of 10 years, and of a case of sudden death of a middle-aged wrestler. Sections V, VI, and VII have been included because they throw light upon the significance of blunt trauma to the chest.

Section IX deals with the problem of *congenital* anomalies of the coronary arteries, another potential cause of death of seemingly healthy persons. Section X contains the description of autopsy findings of a young man who after a 12-mile cross-country race died from *myocarditis.* Although myocarditis is a frequent clinical occurrence, sudden death associated with physical exertion due to inflammatory involvement of the myocardium is less frequent than would be expected considering the overall incidence of inflammatory involvement of the heart, primary or secondary. The probable explanation is that most subjects thus afflicted feel ill and are disinclined to participate in athletic activities.

Section XI by T. N. JAMES, P. FROGGATT, and T. K. MARSHALL focuses attention to the fact that cardiac lesions, even if they are very small in extent, may be fatal if they *cause damage to the conduction system*, a finding in agreement with observations by WOLF and BING [6] and by SCHMIDT *et al.* [5]. The accounts by PUGH of '*Deaths from Exposure* on Four Inns Walking Competition,' and by SCHRIER *et al.* on 'Nephropathy Associated with *Heat Stress and Exercise*' (Sections XII and XIII) emphasize the role played by environmental influences as well as by the involvement of extra-cardiac systems. The scope of adjustibility to training of thermo-regulation in normal subjects has been demonstrated by S. ROBINSON [4]. PUGH *et al.* [2] presented evidence on the remarkable ability of Channel swimmers to maintain core temperatures during prolonged immersion in cold water.

Sections XIV, XV, and XVI deal with 3 rare *post-mortem* findings in cases of the kind discussed in this monograph: one of *subaortic stenosis*, one of *rupture of the ascending aorta*, and one of *aortic hypoplasia.* That the latter condition may be related to the occurrence of sudden death of athletes was pointed out by us 30 years ago (XVI). The validity of our assertion was corroborated in an editorial article in the Lancet of February 22, 1969.

Congenital anomalies of the heart do not invariably cause trouble. J. H. CURRENS and PAUL D. WHITE [1] reported on the findings at the autopsy of the famous marathon runner Clarence DeMar who died from a malignant abdominal tumor at the age of 71. The caliber of DeMar's coronary arteries was exceptionally large. The authors suggest that this great athlete's endowment for long-distance running may have been due in part to the good blood supply of his myocardium thus engendered.

Sections XVII and XVIII emphasize the role that *genetic* factors may play in the timing as well as in the establishing of the pathological bases of cardiac seizures [3,7].

Acknowledgement

We wish to thank the editors of J.A.M.A., the 'Lancet', the 'Annals of Internal Medicine', the 'Archives of Internal Medicine' and of the 'American Journal of Cardiology' for their courtesy in granting permission to include the material in Sections I, VII, XI, XIII, XVII and XVIII.

References

1   CURRENS, H. and WHITE, D.: Half a century of running, clinical, physiologic, and autopsy findings in the case of Clarence DeMar ('Mr. Marathon'). New Engl. J. Med. *265:* 988-993 (1969).

2   PUGH, L. G. C. E.; EDHOLM, O. G.; FOX, R. H.; WOLFF, H. S.; HERVEY, G. R.; HAMMOND, W. H.; TANNER, J. M., and WHITEHOUSE, R. H.: A physiological study of Channel swimming. Clin. Sci. *19:* 257-273 (1960).

3   JOKL, E.: Sudden non-traumatic death associated with physical exertion in identical twins. Acta genet. med. gemellol. *1954:* 245.

4   ROBINSON, S.: Training, acclimatization and heat tolerance. Canad. med. Ass. J. *96:* 795-799 (1967).

5   SCHMIDT, A. P.; CONNOLLY, D. C., and TITUS, J. L.: Complete heart block due to inflammatory lesion of conductive system. Mayo Clinic Proc. *44:* 169-175 (1969).

6   WOLF, P. L. and BING, R.: The smallest tumor which causes sudden death: J. amer. med. Ass. *194:* 674-675 (1965).

7   GIKNIS, F. L.; HOLT, D. E.; WHITEMAN, H. W.; SINGH, M. D.; BENCHIMOL, E., and DIMOND, E. G.: Myocardial Infarction in Twenty-Year-Old Identical Twins. Medicine and Sport, vol. 5, pp. 159-165 (Karger, Basel 1971).

Medicine and Sport, vol. 5: Exercise and Cardiac Death, pp. 1-4
(Karger, Basel 1971)

Asymptomatic Cardiac Disease Causing Sudden Death in Association with Physical Activity

E. Jokl and T. J. McClellan

We present the results of 4 autopsies conducted on persons who died in association with exercise. In each instance the cause of death was cardiac disease which had developed silently and without impairment of physical fitness. The issue is of major relevance to pathology in general. It has special implications for sports-, aviation-, military-, insurance-, and industrial medicine [1-5].

In the first case the cause of death was coronary athero- and arteriosclerosis with myocardial involvement; in the second a congenital anomaly of the coronary arteries; in the third chronic myocarditis; and in the fourth cardiac tumor. The relative frequency with which the above conditions are found *post-mortem* in cases of the kind under reference differs considerably as has been pointed out elsewhere [6-9].

Case 1. A well-trained athlete, age 45, died a few minutes after participating in a wrestling match. Autopsy revealed advanced coronary athero- and arterio-sclerosis, scar tissue scattered throughout the myocardium. A fresh thrombus obstructed the left descending branch of the coronary artery (cp. p. 82).

Case 2. A 16-year-old high school boy dropped dead while playing basketball. Autopsy revealed an enlarged and hypertrophied heart weighing 600 g (normal weight of hearts of 16-year-old boys is 220-280 g). Both coronary arteries were underdeveloped. The left coronary artery arose anomalously from the right anterior aortic sinus. Widespread spotty myocardial degeneration was present (cp. p. 91).

Case 3. A 25-year-old athlete collapsed and died a few minutes after completing a 12-mile cross-country race. $2\frac{1}{2}$ months ago he had contracted a gonorrheal infection of the urethra. Autopsy revealed numerous fibromatous islands in the myocardium and infiltrates containing histiocytes and plasma cells. There was marked hyalinization of the intima of the smaller branches of the coronary arteries (cp. p. 99), [10].

Case 4. While playing at home, a 7-year-old girl suddenly fell unconscious and died 15 min. later. Autopsy revealed a large intracardiac mass attached to the left ventricle (fig. 1). Histologically the tumor was composed entirely of fibrous tissue (fig. 2 and 3).

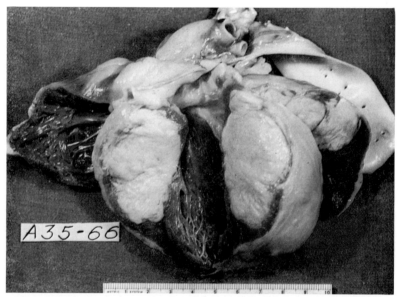

1

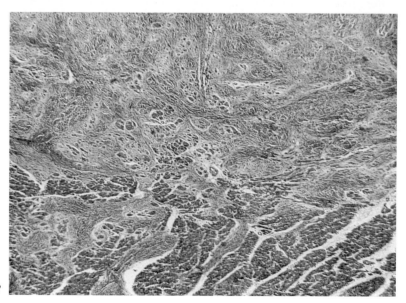

2

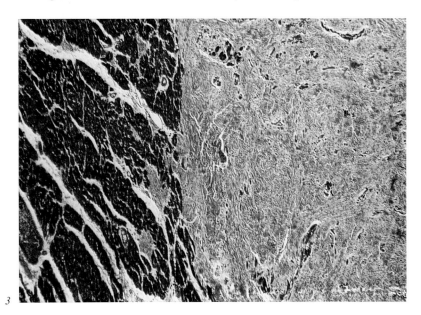

3

Discussion and Conclusions

The foregoing report is concerned with four cases of sudden cardiac death during exercise of seemingly healthy subjects. In the first, autopsy revealed coronary athero- and arterio-sclerosis with myocardial involvement; in the second, a congenital anomaly of the coronary arteries; in the third, chronic myocarditis; in the fourth, an intra-cardiac tumor. The evidence raises the questions of the pathogenesis of cardiac symptoms and of the mechanisms responsible for the onset of fatal seizures of the kind under reference [11-15].

Summary

Potentially fatal cardiac disease may manifest itself first by the terminal collapse. The preceding natural history of illnesses belonging to the nosological category thus identified is distinguished by the absence of symptoms and by unimpaired physical fitness. Four cases are described, each representing a diagnostic entity of the kind under reference.

References

1 CLUVER, E. H. and JOKL, E.: Sudden death of a rugby international after a test game. Amer. Heart J. *24:* 405-409 (1942).

2 JOKL, E. and McCLELLAN, J. T.: Sudden cardiac death of pilots in flight. Cardiologia. *52:* 210-234 (1968).

3 PONSOLD, A.: Abgang der linken Koronararterie von der Pulmonalis als Ursache plötzlichen Todes. Dtsch. Militärarzt. *4:* 137 (1939).

4 SPILSBURY, B.: Death, sudden and unexpected; British Encyclopedia of Medical Practice, *3:* 565-582 (Butterworth, London 1937).

5 JOKL, E. and MELZER, L.: Acute fatal non-traumatic collapse during work and sport. Sth afr. J. med. Sci. *5:* 4-14 (1940).

6 BRUNNER, D. and JOKL, E.: Physical activity and aging; in Medicine and Sport, *4* (Karger, Basel-New York 1969).

7 McCLELLAN, J. T. and JOKL, E.: Congenital anomalies of coronary arteries as cause of sudden death associated with physical exertion. Amer. J. clin. Path. *50:* 229-233 (1968).

8 JOKL, E.: Sudden non-traumatic death associated with physical exertion, with special reference to drowning. Minerva med. *4:* 11-34 (1964).

9 JAMES, T. N.; FROGGATT, P. and MARSHALL, T. K.: Sudden death in young athletes. Ann. intern. Med. *5:* 1013-1021 (1967).

10 JOKL, E.: Plötzlicher Sporttod durch Myokarditis bei Gonorrhoe. Z. Haut-Geschlkr. XIII, *7:* 212-213 (1952).

11 Why did he die? Editorial: J. amer. med. Ass. *1964:* 130-131.

12 Report of the committee on the effect of strain and trauma on the heart and great vessels. Mod. Conc. cardiovasc. Dis., *5:* 793-798 (1963).

13 KAGAN, A.; LIVSIC, A. M.; STERNBY, N., and VIHERT, A. M.: Coronary artery thrombosis and the acute attack of coronary heart disease. Lancet, *December 7:* 1199-1202 (1968).

14 WOLF, P. L. and BING, R.: The smallest tumor which causes sudden death. J. amer. med. Ass. *194:* 674-675 (1965).

15 Symposium on work and the heart. Amer. J. Cardiol. *6:* 729-730 (1964).

Authors' address: University of Kentucky, *Lexington, KY 40506* (USA)

Medicine and Sport, vol. 5: Exercise and Cardiac Death, pp. 5–18
(Karger, Basel 1971)

Acute Fatal Non-Traumatic Collapse
During Work and Sport

E. Jokl and L. Melzer

This paper is a critical analysis of well-studied cases of acute non-traumatic collapse during work or sport. The object of this investigation was to ascertain whether physical strain could lead to fatal collapse due to pathological processes other than those so far known to be responsible for sudden death [Lisa, 1939; Lisa and Hart, 1939].

Table I represents a survey of 43 cases of acute fatal non-traumatic collapse during sport and work which the writers were able to collect from the more recent literature. Older communications such as that of Laurence [1860] did not, for obvious reasons, receive consideration. Only cases in which a complete autopsy was performed were included. It is necessary to emphasise this point, as numerous papers discuss the question under review in general terms without referring to proper pathological investigations [Schürmann, 1939].

The writers have not included cases of heatstroke, which they had ample opportunity to study in native workers in the Transvaal Gold Mines. No consideration has been given in this paper to another interesting problem closely related to the subject matter of this survey, namely to the question of sudden 'exhaustive' deaths of mentally disordered persons. The latter question has been reviewed by Pende [1928], Bamford and Bean [1932], Derby [1933], Davidson [1934], Stefan [1935], and Shulack [1938].

Table I

No.	Occurrence of death	Autopsy findings	Final diagnosis	Author
1	Cutting wood	Advanced coronary sclerosis. Brown atrophy and fibrosis of heart muscles.	Coronary insufficiency	HOLZMANN and WUHRMANN
2	Carrying heavy luggage	Fibrosis of heart muscle. Coronary atheromatosis.	Coronary insufficiency	STEPHENSON
3	Manual labour on hot day	Aortitis syphilitica. Right coronary artery blocked.	Coronary occlusion	BRACK
4	Walking 10 miles	Atherosclerosis of aorta, including valv s. Ostium of right coronary artery almost occluded.	Coronary insufficiency	KORBSCH
5	Playing football	Lipoidosis of intima of aorta, aortic valves and coronary artery.	Coronary insufficiency	BRACK
6	Tennis tournament	Haemopericardium, rupture of ascending aorta. Tear in intima of aorta, obviously older than tear in adventitia. Four days interval between collapse and death.	Rupture of aorta Aneurysma dissecans Endarteritis	HARDAWAY and GREEN
7	Running in a race	Ruptured aneurysm in tuberculous pulmonary cavity.	Ruptured aneurysm	BRACK
8	Walking to college (examination day)	Heart 3 times size of fist. Weight: 750 g. Inflammatory and degenerative processes in myocardium.	Myocarditis	WERCKMEISTER
9	Cross-country race	Inflammatory vegetations on aortic valve, distension of mitral ostium. Hypertrophy and dilatation of heart.	Endocarditis	SCHÖNEBERG
10	Bathing in sea	Coronary sclerosis. Sclerosis of kidneys. Fatty degeneration of myocardium.	Coronary sclerosis Myocardial degeneration	GRAVENHORST
11	Running mile race	Aortic stenosis. Chronic endocarditis. Organised thrombus in right branch of artery.	Coronary occlusion	SCHÖNEBERG

Table I (continued)

No.	Occurence of death	Autopsy findings	Final diagnosis	Author
12	Riding bicycle after heavy wo k (digging a drain)	Extreme stenosis of aortic orifice which was almost totally occluded. Marked calcification of cusps. Pulmonary tuberculosis. No histological findings in myocardium reported.	Aortic stenosis (state of myocardium?)	CAMPBELL
13	Military drill	Considerable hypertrophy of left heart with dilation. Mitral regurgitation.	Coronary insufficiency	SCHÖNEBERG
14	Walking	Extreme calcification of aortic valves. Aortic ostium narrowed. Hypertrophy of left ventricle.	Sclerosis and stenosis of aortic valves	MARVIN and SULLIVAN
15	Carrying heavy weights	Advanced fatty degeneration of heart muscle.	Myocardial degeneration	WILDE
16	Riding a bicycle	Chronic degeneration of heart muscle. Calcification of coronary vessels.	Coronary insufficiency	SCHÖNEBERG
17	Running 3,000 m	Superior portion of ascending aorta dilated. Intima roughened, numerous whitish scars. Aortic wall thickened. Yellow spots in media. Coronary ostia greatly narrowed. Lumina greatly decreased.	Mesaortitis luetica Coronary insufficiency	LACHMUND
18	Military drill	Degeneration of heart muscle. Chronic ulcerative endocarditis. Aortic stenosis.	Myocardial degeneration	SCHÖNEBERG
19	Military drill	Thrombus in branch of right coronary artery. Endocarditis of mitral valve.	Coronary thrombosis	W. SCHMIDT
20	Mile race	Extreme stenosis of aortic ostium. Hypertrophy and dilatation of left ventricle.	Coronary insufficiency	SCHÖNEBERG
21	Walking	Extreme sclerosis and stenosis of coronary artery.	Coronary insufficiency	NYLIN

Table I (continued)

No.	Occurrence of death	Autopsy findings	Final diagnosis	Author
22	Walking, after considerable exertion	Two independent organised infarcts in left ventricle. Coronary artery blocked by thrombus.	Coronary thrombosis	GOEDVOLK
23	Skipping after lunch	Congenital absence of left coronary artery.	Coronary insufficiency	SPILSBURY
24	Start for sprinting race	Ruptured aneuryms of ramus comm. ant. art. cerebr.	Ruptured cerebral aneurysm	KIRCH
25	Cranking motor car handle for 2 min.	Extensive sclerosis in sinus Valsalvae and aorta. Marked hypertrophy and dilatation of left and dilatation of right ventricle. Interval of 12 weeks between strain and death.	Degeneration of myocardium	WHITE and EARLE-GLENDY
26	Cross-country race	Left coronary artery originates from pulmonary artery.	Coronary insufficiency	PONSOLD
27	Heavy industrial labour (Jack hammer)	Left coronary artery originates from pulmonary artery.	Coronary insufficiency	RUBBERT
28	Hunting on horseback	Advanced atheromatosis of coronary arteries. Necrotic areas in myocardium.	Coronary insufficiency	LEPEL
29	Piloting passenger aeroplane	Coronary thrombosis.	Coronary thrombosis	BENSON
30	Industrial manual work	Advanced coronary sclerosis and atheromatosis.	Coronary insufficiency (syphilis?)	DURCK
31	Carrying heavy stones	Coronary thrombosis.	Coronary thrombosis (syphilis?)	Cases from Medico-Legal Institute of Berlin University, reported by HALLERMANN
32	Swimming	Left descending branch of coronary artery blocked by thick atheromatous patch.	Coronary occlusion	
33	Pushing a heavily loaded wheelbarrow uphill	Aneurysm of apex of heart. Occlusion of left branch of coronary artery.	Coronary insufficiency	

Table I (continued)

No.	Occurrence of death	Autopsy findings	Final diagnosis	Author
34	Carrying furniture	Extreme degree of narrowing of left branch of coronary artery.	Coronary insufficiency	
35	Lifting a heavy weight	Necrotic area in left ventricle, fatty degeneration of myocardium, narrowing of lumen of coronary artery.	Degeneratio cordis	Cases from Medico-Legal Institute
36	Lifting heavy couch	Myocardial degeneration, narrowing of lumen of coronary artery.	Degeneratio cordis, coronary insufficiency	of Berlin University, reported by
37	Transporting heavy goods	Rupture of myocardium within necrotic area.	Rupture of heart	HALLERMANN
38	Butcher, killing animal with 25-lb hammer	Rupture of aneurysm of coronary artery into pericardium.	Ruptured cardiac aneurysm	
39	Beating carpet	Interstitial myocarditis.	Myocarditis	FIEBACH
40	Military drill	Old endocarditis, chronic leptomeningitis. Oedema of brain.	Serous inflammation of vascular endothelia	
41	Athletics	Dilatation of heart. Lymphatic tissues increased. Chronic leptomeningitis.	Not clearly established. Death believed be due to vascular disease.	
42	Walking (first-class athlete)	(Hereditary abnormality. Sister and uncle had died under similar circumstances.) Old endocarditis. Oedema of brain. Chronic leptomeningitis. Stomach greatly distended with food.	Not clearly established. Death believed to be due to vascular disease. Cause of terminal collapse	E. MÜLLER
43	Physical exertion	Old inflammatory reactions on aortic valves. Hyperplasia of lymphatic tissue. Oedema of brain, chronic leptomeningitis. Marked impressiones digitatae. Infiltration of lymphocytes around small blood vessels.	Unexplained (circulatory system seriously diseased)	

Additional Material

The authors surveyed all reports of autopsies made on cases of acute fatal non-traumatic collapse during work and sport which were investigated at the South African Police Medico-Legal Laboratories in Johannesburg between 1934 and 1939. From a total of 6,370 autopsies, they collected 20 cases, a 21st case being added from a previous observation made by JOKL [1933].

Table II gives a survey of the essential facts of these cases.

Table II

No.	Description and age	Occurrence of death	Autopsy (excerpts)	Final diagnosis
1	Male: 40	Chopping wood	Haemorrhage into pericardial sac. Aorta dilated. Areas of softening present. Rupture of ascending aorta.	Rupture of aorta
2	Male: 58	At work	Arterio-sclerosis. Pericardial sac filled with blood clot. Dilatation of aortic arch. Rupture of aorta in ascending part of arch. Arterio-sclerotic changes in kidney.	Rupture of aorta
3	Male: 45	After coming to surface from under-ground work in gold mine	Left lung very adherent. Tuber-culous cavity in apex. Ruptured blood vessel in cavity, profuse haemorrhage into lung. Both lungs fibrosed and emphyse-matous.	Rupture of blood vessel in tuberculous lung
4	Male: 23	During under-ground work in gold mine	Extensive subdural and basal haemorrhage of brain. Ventricles filled with blood. Rupture of aneurysm of left posterior communicating artery.	Rupture of cerebral aneurysm
5	Male: 55	While gardening	Aortic valve incompetent. Atheromatosis of aorta and coronary arteries. Hypertrophy of muscle. Adherent pericardium.	Myocarditis

Table II (continued)

No.	Discription and age	Occurrence of death	Autopsy (excerpts)	Final diagnosis
6	Male: 35	While riding a bicycle	Heart dilated and hypertrophied. Aortic valve incompetent, cusps hard and thickened. Mitral valve incompetent. Coronary arteries sclerosed.	Coronary insufficiency
7	Male: 49	During work	Large basal haemorrhage of brain. Ruptured aneurysm of anterior cerebral artery.	Rupture of cerebral aneurysm
8	Male: 48	While playing bowls	Sclerosis of coronary vessels.	Coronary insufficiency
9	Male: 25	While playing football	Heart dilated. Inflammatory vegetations on cusps of mitral valve.	Infective endocarditis and myocarditis
10	Male: 60	While cycling	Hypertrophy and dilatation of heart, mainly on left side. Endocardium thickened and opaque. Patchy fibrosis of myocardium, particularly of papillary muscles. Considerable atheromatosis of coronary vessels. Atheromatosis of aorta, paricularly of abdominal aorta.	Coronary insufficiency Myocarditis
11	Female: 43	While scrubbing the floor	Left ventricle dilated and hypertrophied. Syphilitic aortitis. Saccular aneurysm in thoracic aorta. Sac filled with laminated clot. Rupture of sac into oesophagus.	Rupture of aortic aneurysm
12	Male: 64	Collapsed during swimming and died shortly afterwards	Hypertrophy and dilatation of left ventricle. Atheromatous changes in descending aorta. Fatty infiltration of heart muscle.	Chronic myocarditis
13	Male: 40	While walking quickly	Rupture of aortic aneurysm. Arterio-sclerosis of aorta.	Rupture of aortic aneurysm
14	Male: 40	Collapsed and died after a dance	Fibrosis of heart muscle, especially of papillary muscle. Large calcified atheromatous spots in aorta.	Chronic myocarditis

Table II (continued)

No.	Description and age	Occurrence of death	Autopsy (excerpts)	Final diagnosis
15	Male: 35	Died during work	Rupture of a aortic aneurysm.	Rupture of aortic aneurysm
16	Female: 55	Collapsed during work	Rupture of aortic aneurysm.	Rupture of aortic aneurysm
17	Male: 52	Died during cricket game	Small flaccid heart. Extreme sclerosis of coronary vessels.	Coronary insufficiency
18	Male: 20	Died during football match	Haemorrhage into pericardial sac. Small flaccid heart. Rupture of right ventricle. Coronary arteries almost blocked through endarteritic vegetations.	Rupture of right ventricle
19	Male: 33	Died during football match	Extreme sclerosis of coronary arteries. Stomach distended with food.	Coronary insufficiency
20	Male: 34	Died during football match	Extreme sclerosis of coronary artery. Chronic myocarditis. Atheromatosis of aorta.	Coronary insufficiency
21	Female: 16	Died during dance	Congenital sub-aortic stenosis. Hypertrophy of left ventricle. Marked myocardial degeneration.	Sub-aortic stenosis Myodegeneratio cordis

Results

In the above instances of death, autopsy revealed the presence of pathological conditions, in the great majority of long standing and of great severity. *Not one instance was encountered in which death could be regarded as due to the effects of extreme exertion on a previously healthy heart.* It is significant that there is no case in our list in which death occurred during a physical performance longer and more intense than that in which the deceased had usually indulged.

Of the three 'master systems of the body,' the circulatory, the respiratory and the nervous [SPILSBURY, 1937], one of which is invariably involved in cases of sudden death, the circulatory system is by far the most important in regard to fatal collapse during work and sport. *In our own cases, the cause of death was without exception found to be connected with the circulatory system*, one of the following conditions being responsible for the fatal collapse: coronary arterial disease; aneurysm of aorta, cerebral arteries, heart; inflammatory disease of the heart muscle, degenerative disease of the heart muscle; rupture of the aorta, and rupture of heart muscle. In a few reported instances in which the central nervous system was involved [MÜLLER, 1939], it was found that the primary cause of death lay with the vascular system.

Functional Pathology

The following three physiological reactions must be understood for the analysis of the functional mechanisms immediately responsible for breakdowns of the circulatory system during exercise.

1. *The rise of arterial systolic blood pressure* which normally accompanies physical exertion [McCURDY and McKENZIE, 1928; ELDAHL, 1933]. This rise of blood pressure is directly responsible for fatal ruptures of blood vessels affected by congenital, arteriosclerotic, inflammatory and especially syphilitic and tuberculous processes (cf cases 6, 7, 24 in table I and 1, 2, 3, 4, 7, 11, 13, 15, 16 and 18 in table II).

2. *Expiratory effort* against the closed glottis (Valsalva) such as is invariably associated with muscular work, causes considerable stress, even on the healthy heart. Rising intrathoracic pressure obstructs the normal venous return to the right auricle, causing a sharp increase of venous pressure [BAUMANN, 1935]. At the same time, reflexes from the carotid sinuses and aortic arch lead to an immediate rise of arterial pressure [HEYMANS, 1938; BÜRGER, 1933]. Simultaneously, oxygen saturation of the capillary blood decreases rapidly, more so during or immediately after exercise [MATTHES, 1935]. That means that the heart with its blood supply markedly diminished for at least a short period, is forced to work against increased resistance. It is not surprising, therefore, that systematic tests carried out on apparently healthy athletes, students and pilots, revealed various abnormal reactions during or after expiratory effort. BORST [1934] as well as SCHLOMKA [1937] have noted syncope, displacement of the

pace-maker of the heart beat, auricular block, ventricular automatism, auricular and ventricular extrasystoles, heart pauses lasting several seconds and abnormal changes of frequency of the heart beat. Electro-cardiographic studies suggest that at least some of the physiological as well as abnormal circulatory reactions during or after expiratory efforts are due to an acute impairment of coronary blood supply. If cardiac reactions of undoubtedly abnormal character occur in apparently healthy young men, how much greater must the danger be to the hearts of diseased individuals during expiratory pressing?

3. *The gastro-coronary reflex:* The practical importance of this pheno-menon was stressed by G. BERGMANN [1936] at whose clinic it was investi-gated [DIETRICH and SCHWIEGK, 1933, 1934]. If intragastric pressure is raised, especially in the proximal portion of the stomach, a nervous reflex is elicited, leading to acute coronary constriction and consequently to impairment of blood and oxygen supply of the heart muscle. Since the oxygen requirements of the myocardium are considerably increased during exertion, this reflex must produce unfavourable effects in diseased hearts. It has been shown by JARISCH and LILJESTRAND [1927], that even the normal circulatory system works less economically if the stomach is distended and the inadvisability of performing strenuous exercise after meals is generally recognised. The writers have attached significance to the obser-vation that marked distension of the stomach with food was found in a number of their cases.

Rise of systolic blood pressure whether brought about by muscular activity or by expiratory effort, interferes with the normal venous return to the heart. This and the effects of the gastro-coronary reflex tax the functional integrity of the myocardium to the utmost; the heart can escape damage only if its reserve powers are adequate, i.e. if the myocardial tissue is healthy. In subjects suffering from arteriosclerosis, from inflam-matory or degenerative coronary disease or from insufficient blood supply of the myocardium, exercise may thus spell disaster.

Some Practical Aspects of the Problem

Many people have a markedly diseased circulatory system but are unaware of their condition. Such individuals may even be outstanding performers as industrial workers or as competitive athletes. Cases 6, 9, 11,

17 and 24 in table I and 9 and 18 in table II serve as typical examples. Case 18, which refers to a young first league footbal player was particularly impressive since during the 3 years preceding his death the victim had been one of the most prominent soccer players in a large town, and never complained of any distress and was generally regarded as extraordinarily fit.

JOKL [1933, 1935, 1936] has reported a number of cases of athletes with severely diseased hearts who were successful in open athletic competitions. One of the best marathon runners of the British Empire, a first league football player and a sprinting champion were studied in detail, had aortic regurgitation and mitral stenosis [JOKL and SUZMAN, 1940]. HEIL-MANN [1938] reported on the case of a soldier of 23 years of age, in whom a routine X-ray examination led to the discovery of a large aneurysm of the aorta. No clinical symptoms whatsoever were present and the patient had successfully participated in sport and athletics, including long-distance walks and races.

It must be emphasised that the degree of 'fitness' as measured by athletic efficiency is certainly no reliable indication of the presence or absence of organic changes of the circulatory system.

A point of interest is that we have not yet encountered a single subject with *valvular* disease of the heart, in whom the *myocardium* and *coronary system* were healthy, dying suddenly during work or sport. In view of the fact that SPILSBURY [1937] states that aortic incompetence occasionally causes sudden death, it is noteworthy that, as far as the writers know, no case histories of fatal collapse due to uncomplicated aortic incompetence during work or sport have been published. On the contrary, there are numerous instances of aortic incompetence in successful athletes and industrial workers [JOKL, 1935]. Attention is also drawn to cases of the kind observed by SCHMIDT [1938] and by HARDAWAY and GREEN [1935] (6 in table II) in which small and apparently insignificant histopathological foci of disease, which had neither impaired physical well-being nor made first-class athletic performances impossible, were responsible for fatal collapses during exertion.

'A miniature or inconspicuous lesion may be the main factor in such a type of death with the result that sometimes painstaking search is required to find it. Such cases are not only of scientific interest but they may have far-reaching forensic implications' [HELWIG and WILHELMY, 1939].

Finally, mention should be made of the extreme rarity of acute collapse during exertion due to iliac emboli. Iliac emboli are responsible for one of the most typical causes of pathological breakdowns in racing horses.

Summary

Among 6,370 cases on which autopsies were carried out at the South African Police Medico-Legal Laboratories between 1934 and 1939, there were 20 instances of acute fatal breakdowns during work and sport. Another 43 cases were collected from literature. Only cases where an autopsy was performed were considered. No case was encountered of a previously healthy individual having died suddenly from excessive exertion. In all cases of death during sport or work, autopsy revealed the presence of one or more of the following diseases of the circulatory system: coronary arterial disease, aneurysm of aorta, cerebral arteries, pulmonary arteries; inflammatory disease of the heart muscle; degenerative disease of the heart muscle; rupture of heart muscle, and rupture of aorta.

References

ABRAHAMS, A.: Athletics. Brit. Encyclopedia med. Practice (London, 1936).

BAETZNER, W.: Sport und Arbeitschaden (Thieme, Leipzig, 1936).

BAMFORD, C. and BEAN, H.: J. ment. Sci. *78:* 353 (1932).

BARBER, H.: Brit. med. J. *i:* 433 (1938).

BAUMANN, H.: Klin. Wschr. *1:* 386 (1935).

BENSON, O.: J. Aviation Med. *8:* 81 (1937).

BERGMANN, G., v.: Funktionelle Pathologie (Springer, Berlin 1936).

BOAS, E. P.: J. amer. med. Ass. *112:* 1887 (1939).

BORST, W.: Klin. Wschr. *11:* 1921 (1934).

BRACK, E.: Med. Welt. *1:* 932 (1934).

BRAHDY, L. and KAHN, S.: Trauma and Disease (Lea and Febiger, Philadelphia 1937).

BÜRGER, M.: Blutkreislauf, in Norm. u. Path. Physiologie der Leibesübungen (Barth, Leipzig 1933).

CAMPBELL, M.: Supplement to Marvin and Sullivan's paper. Amer. Heart J. *10:* 705 (1935).

DAVIDSON, G. M.: Amer. J. Psychiat. *91:* 41 (1934).

DERBY, I. M.: Psychiat. Quart. *7:* 436 (1933).

DIETRICH, A. and SCHWIEGK, S.: Z. klin. Med. *125:* 967 (1933).

DIETRICH, A. and SCHWIEGK, S.: Dtsch. med. Wschr. *26:* 967 (1934).

ELDAHL, A.: Arbeitsphysiol. *7:* 437 (1933).

FIEBACH, R.: Virchows Arch. path. Anat. *233:* 57 (1921).

GOEDVOLK, C.: Personal communication (1935).

GRAVENHORST: Der Tod im Wasser als versicherungsrechtliches Problem. Hefte zur Unfallsheilkunde *20:* (Vogel, Berlin 1937).

HARDAWAY, R. N. and GREEN, M. M.: Amer. Heart J. *10:* 385 (1935).

HARTLEY, P. and LLEWELLYN, G. F.: Brit. med. J. *i:* 657 (1939).

HEILMANN, P.: Dtsch. Militärarzt *9:* 402 (1938).

HELLERMANN, W.: Der plötzliche Herztod bei Kranzgefässerkrankungen (F. Enke, Stuttgart 1938).

HELWIG, C. F. and WILHELMY, E. W.: Ann. intern. Med. *13:* 107 (1939).

HEYMANS, C.: New Engl. J. Med. *219:* 147 (1938).

HOLZMANN, M. and WUHRMANN, F.: Dtsch. med. Wschr. *62:* 685 (1936).

HUEPPE, F.: Leibesübungen, *1:* 143 (1935).

JARISCH and LILJESTRAND, G.: Skand. Arch. Physiol. *51:* 235 (1927).

JOKL, E.: Schweiz. med. Wschr. 49, *2:* 1278 (1933).

JOKL, E.: The Leech *6:* 35 (1935).

JOKL, E.: Zusammenbrüche beim Sport (Manz, Wien 1936).

JOKL, E. and PARADE, W.: Med. Klin. *29:* 1070 (1933).

JOKL, E. and SUZMAN, M. M.: J. amer. med. Ass. *114:* 467 (1940).

KIRCH, E.: Verh. dtsch. Ges. inn. Med. *47:* 73 (1935).

KLAUS, E. J.: Dtsch. Arch. klin. Med. *181:* 275 (1937).

KNOLL, E.: Dtsch. med. Wschr. 63, *2:* 1483 (1937).

KORBSCH, L.: Dtsch. mil.-ärztl. Z. *32:* 9 (1914).

LACHMUND, H.: Leibesübungen *1:* 635 (1930).

LAURENCE, J. Z.: Brit. med. J. *i:* 376 (1860).

LEPEL: Dtsch. Militärarzt *3:* 524 (1938).

LEWIS, Th.: The soldiers' heart and the effort syndrome (H. M. Stat. Off., London 1918).

LISA, J. R.: Ann. intern. Med. *12:* 1968 (1939).

LISA, J. R. and HART, F.: Arch. intern. Med. *64:* 48 (1939).

LORENTZ, H.: Der Gesundheitswert der Sportarten (Barth, Stuttgart 1938).

MARVIN, H. M. and SULLIVAN, F.: Amer. Heart J. *10:* 705 (1935).

MASTER, A. M.: J. amer. med. Ass. *113:* 440 (1939).

MASTER, A. M.; JAFFE, H. L. and DACK, S.: J. amer. med. Ass. *112:* 1020 (1939).

McCURDY, H. J. and McKENZIE, R. T.: The physiology of exercise (Lea and Febiger, Philadelphia 1928).

MATTHES, K.: Verh. dtsch. Ges. Kreislforsch. *6:* 139 (1935).

MÜLLER, E.: Virchows Arch. path. Anat. *303:* 588 (1939).

MURCH, H.: Münch. med. Wschr. *78:* 627 (1931).

NYLIN, G.: J. amer. med. Ass. *109:* 1333 (1937).

NYLIN, G.: Acta med. scand. *78:* 64 (1938).

PATERSON, J. G.: J. amer. med. Ass. *112:* 895 (1939).

PENDE, N.: Constitutional inadequacies (Lea and Febiger, Philadelphia 1928).

PONSOLD, A.: Dtsch. Militärarzt *4:* 201 (1939).

RUBBERT, H.: Beitr. path. Anat. allg. Path. *122:* 98 (1936).

SCHLOMKA, G.: Luftfhrt. med. Abh. *1:* 169 (1937).

SCHMIDT, W.: Dtsch. Militärarzt *3:* 351 (1938).

SCHÖNEBERG, H.: Dtsch. med. Wschr. *19:* 1, 17 (1936).

SHULACK, N. R.: Psychiat. Quart. *12:* 282 (1938).

SCHÜRMANN: Dtsch. Militärarzt *4:* 408 (1939).

SPICER, F.W.: Trauma and internal disease (Lippincott, Philadelphia 1939).

SPILSBURY, B.: Brit. Encyclopaedia med. Practice, vol. 3 (Butterworth, London 1937).

STEFAN, H.: Dtsch. med. Wschr. 60, *2:* 1550 (1924).

STEFAN, H.: Z. ges. Neurol. Psychiat. *152:* 480 (1935).
STEPHENSON, G. E.: Newcastle med. J. *9:* 208 (1929).
WERCKMEISTER, R.: Zbl. allg. Path. path. Anat. *53:* 11 (1932).
WHITE, P. D. and GLENDY, R. E.: (quoted by Brahdy and Kahn.)
WILDE, A.: Med. Klin. *19:* 247 (1923).

Authors' address: University of Kentucky, *Lexington, KY 40506* (USA)

Medicine and Sport, vol. 5: Exercise and Cardiac Death, pp. 19–24
(Karger, Basel 1971)

Mechanisms Involved in Acute Fatal Nontraumatic Collapse Associated with Physical Exertion

E. Jokl and M. M. Suzman

The problem of acute, fatal, nontraumatic collapse during sport and work has been investigated by Jokl and Melzer [1940] and by Cluver and Jokl [1941]. An analysis of 66 cases, in which clinical data as well as complete autopsy reports were available, revealed that collapse associated with exertion is almost invariably due to circulatory disease of long standing. In no case in which death occurred in connection with physical exertion was the subject found at autopsy to be free of serious disease.

Pathologic Findings

The following conditions, arranged in order of frequency, were found at autopsy: (1) coronary artery disease; (2) acute coronary occlusion; (3) degenerative disease of heart muscle; (4) ruptured aneurysm of aorta; (5) inflammatory disease of heart muscle; (6) ruptured aneurysm of cerebral arteries, usually congenital; (7) rupture of heart; (8) rupture of congenitally diseased aorta; (9) developmental abnormalities of the heart; (10) developmental hypoplasia of entire arterial system.

Thus, of the 3 'master systems of the body' [Spilsbury, 1937], the circulatory, the respiratory, and the nervous, the circulatory is by far the most frequently involved in fatal nontraumatic collapse associated with work and sport.

Pathophysiologic Considerations

For the analysis of the functional mechanisms involved in the break-down of the diseased circulatory system during exertion, the following physiologic reactions must be considered:

1. The biphasic reaction of the arterial blood pressure to exercise. Physiologically arterial blood pressure rises during exercise and drops below the initial level during the rest period following exertion. We therefore speak of the 'biphasic reaction to exercise.' Whenever the autopsy revealed that death had been due to rupture of diseased blood vessels, it was ascertained that the first symptoms of the collapse which preceded death had set in *during* the muscular effort. As muscular exertion is accompanied by a rise of arterial systolic blood pressure, this physiologic reaction is therefore considered directly responsible for the rupturing of the affected blood vessels.

The phase of elevated blood pressure during exercise is followed by a depression during the rest period *after* the exertion, when the arterial pressure usually drops lower than the initial level. During this 'nega-tive phase,' the significance of which for the coronary blood supply has been stressed by BLUMGART, SCHLESINGER, and DAVIS [1940], there is distinct danger to subjects who suffer from coronary and myocardial disease.

Among our own cases was that of a football player who lost conscious-ness *after* a league match and died 30 min later. At autopsy his heart muscle showed general hypertrophy and advanced fibrosis. Another example is that of a 16-year-old girl who, having collapsed after dancing for 3 hours, died a few minutes later. At autopsy, examination revealed congenital subaortic stenosis, marked hypertrophy of the left ventricle, and advanced myocardial degeneration.

2. Expiratory effort ('Valsalva' phenomenon). We consider that expiratory effort against the closed glottis represents the greatest physiologic stress with which the heart has to cope.

The diffusion of oxygen through the lung may be virtually suspended, and oxygen saturation of the capillary blood consequently decreases rapidly. This decrease has been shown by MATTHES [1935] to be most marked during or immediately after exercise when the oxygen requirements of the tissues are raised. Moreover, the elevated intrathoracic pressure impedes the return of blood to the right auricle, leading to a sharp increase of systemic venous pressure [BAUMANN, 1935]. The diminished output of the right ventricle as well as the greatly increased intrapulmonary pressure seriously interferes with the pulmonary circulation, leading to deficient filling of the left ventricle which through the fluoroscope can be seen to 'beat empty' ('leerschlagen'). Thus, the filling of, and the pressure in, the ascending aorta decrease acutely, and coronary blood flow consequently diminishes sharply. VISSCHER [1939] has drawn attention to what he calls 'the pressure gradient mechanism' on which the coronary blood flow, like any other fluid in an hydraulic system, depends. This pressure gradient, he says, so far as the coronary system is concerned, is measured by the difference in pressure between aorta, and the coronary sinus and right ventricle. As the intra-aortic pressure decreases during expiratory effort, the pressure gradient flattens and coronary blood supply decreases sharply. Thus, myocardial respiration is greatly impaired. Although reflexes from the carotid sinus and aortic arch, in the face of a lowered aortic pressure, usually lead to a rise of *peripheral* arterial pressure due to arteriolar vaso-constriction [BÜRGER, 1935; HEYMANS, 1937], myocardial blood supply is likely to suffer greatly.

The profound pathophysiologic significance of this phase must be viewed in the light of the classic work of SHIPLEY, SHIPLEY and WEARN [1935]. These authors showed that a pathologically hypertrophied heart muscle possesses, per unit of myocardial tissue, a considerably smaller number of capillaries than a normal heart muscle. The area of myocardial tissue supplied by a single capillary, is enlarged in the pathologically hypertrophied heart. It exceeds greatly the equivalent area in the heart of the healthy, though untrained, subject. The richest capillary supply is found in the heart of the trained healthy athlete [PETREN, SJÖSTRAND and SYLVEN, 1936]. This is the reason why the heart of *trained healthy* subjects, whose respiratory tissue requirements are readily satisfied, will practically never be endangered, even in the course of strenuous athletic performances which demand extreme expiratory efforts; whereas, on the other hand, impeded myocardial blood supply implies a considerable risk in *all* situa-tions, in which expiratory efforts against the closed glottis occurs. Exercise represents one of these situations.

In subjects with coronary artery disease, and deficient capillary supply of a hypertrophic myocardium, this physiologic phase therefore often represents a catastrophic event from which the heart may never recover. Sudden death has frequently been encountered in middleaged and, occasionally, in young persons, in the course of physical activities, such as carrying heavy weights, gymnastic exercises, pushing a wheel-barrow, cycling up hill, or wrestling. In the majority of these cases autopsy revealed coronary and myocardial disease.

3. The gastrocoronary reflex. Rise of intragastric pressure, especially, it is claimed, in the proximal portion of the stomach, elicits a reflex constriction of the coronary arterial system. The practical importance of the gastrocoronary reflex was first stressed by G. VON BERGMANN [1936] at whose clinic it had been investigated [DIETRICH and SCHWIEGK, 1933, 1934]. Subsequently, the physiologic and clinical implications of this problem were carefully studied by GILBERT [1939] and GILBERT et al. [1940]. During physical exertion, when the oxygen requirements of the myocardium are considerably increased, the gastrocoronary reflex may result in serious anoxemia in the heart in which the tissue respiration is already impaired by disease. It has been shown by JARISCH and LILJESTRAND [1927] that even the healthy circulation functions less economically if the stomach is distended, a result which represents the scientific basis for the empirical rule that after meals strenuous exercise is inadvisable. We therefore attach significance to the fact that in 7 of our own cases the stomach was found distended with food. Two subjects were known to have taken part in strenuous games immediately after having consumed big meals. When they collapsed, they vomited very large quantities of undigested food, whereafter they experienced temporary symptomatic relief. SPILSBURY [1937] reported the case of a young woman who collapsed while skipping after a meal and died shortly afterward. Autopsy revealed congenital absence of the left branch of the coronary artery. It may be assumed that in this instance too the gastrocoronary reflex had caused a critical reduction of the oxygen supply to the myocardium.

Physical Efficiency and Circulatory Disease

It is remarkable that cardiovascular disease, so serious that it may cause death at any moment, does not necessarily interfere with even an extraordinarily high standard of physical efficiency. JOKL and PARADE [1933] described several cases of athletes with valvular defects. JOKL and SUZMAN [1940] have studied a marathon champion with aortic regurgitation and mitral stenosis. SUZMAN has observed a young wrestler who, in spite of the presence of mitral stenosis with enormous dilation of the heart and signs of congestive cardiac failure with cyanosis, continued, against advice, to take part successfully in wrestling bouts. CLUVER and JOKL [1941] have communicated the case of 'The Iron Man of South African Rugby,' who died a few minutes after a test game in which he excelled in the same way as on innumerable previous occasions. Autopsy revealed a grossly under-developed abdominal aorta, an almost totally degenerated left, and a grossly hypertrophied right kidney, a hypertrophied and degenerated heart muscle, an underdeveloped, partly obliterated, atheromatous coronary artery, and a large thymus gland, which, from the histologic appearance, could be assumed to have been functionally active. This collection of pathologic features must have been present for many years, and yet the 'patient' had been outstanding rugby players during the decade preceding his death. An identical twin brother of the deceased had died a short time before, also during physical exertion (swimming).

We have included in this analysis only *nontraumatic* collapses. No reference is made to the large number of athletic fatalities of traumatic origin, many of which are due to injury to the central nervous system. As an example of this group, JOKL [1941] has recently analyzed a branch of sport (boxing) in which specific athletic traumata are primarily responsible for fatal incidents. With regard to *nontraumatic* fatal collapses during or after effort, the position is entirely different. While normally no conceivable functional strain can cause fatal collapse [SUZMAN and JOKL, 1936], certain diseases, such as those enumerated in this paper, render heart and blood vessels so vulnerable that the physiologic effort associated with physical exertion may overtax their adaptive plasticity.

Summary

The results of an analysis of 66 cases of sudden death from physical exertion are discussed. The pathologic findings are given and interpreted.

A special attempt has been made to clarify the part played by physiologic reactions to exercises, in leading to the fatal breakdown. The following physiologic phenomena have been considered in detail: (1) the biphasic reaction of the arterial blood pressure to exercise, (2) expiratory effort (Valsalva phenomenon), and (3) the gastrocoronary reflex. Attention has been drawn to the fact that even advanced circulatory disease is not necessarily accompanied by a decrease or a low state of physical efficiency.

References

1   ABRAHAMS, A.: Athletics. Brit. Encyclopaedia med. Practice, vol. 2 (London 1936).
2   BERGMANN, G. v.: Funktionelle Pathologie (Springer, Berlin 1936).
3   BLUMGART, H. L.; SCHLESINGER, M. J., and DAVIS, D.: Amer. Heart J. *19:* 1 (1940).
4   BÜRGER, M.: Blutkreislauf, in Norm. u. Path. Physiologie der Leibesübungen (Barth, Leipzig 1933).
5   CLUVER, E. H. and JOKL, E.: Amer. Heart J. *24:* 405 (1942).
6   DIETRICH, A. and SCHWIEGK, S.: Z. klin. Med. *125:* 967 (1933).
7   DIETRICH, A. and SCHWIEGK, S.: Dtsch. med. Wschr. *26:* 967 (1934).
8   GILBERT, N. C.: J. amer. med. Ass. *113:* 1925 (1939).
9   GILBERT, N. C.; FENN, G. K., and LE ROY, G. V.: J. amer. med. Ass. *115:* 1962 (1940).
10   GILBERT, N. C.; LE ROY, G. V., and FENN, G. K.: The effect of distention of abdominal viscera on the blood flow in the circumflex branch of the left coronary artery of the dog. Amer. Heart J. *20:* 519 (1940).
11   HEYMANS, C.: New Engl. J. Med. *219:* 147 (1938).
12   JARISCH and LILJESTRAND, G.: Skand. Arch. Physiol. *51:* 235 (1927).
13   JOKL, E. and PARADE, H. W.: Med. Klin. *32:* (1933).
14   JOKL, E.: The medical aspect of boxing (van Schaik, Pretoria 1941).
15   JOKL, E. and SUZMAN, M. M.: J. amer. med. Ass. *114:* 467 (1940).
16   PETREN, T.; SJÖSTRAND, S., and SYLVEN, B.: Arbeitsphysiol. (1936).
17   SHIPLEY, R.; SHIPLEY, J., and WEARN, J. T.: J. exper. Med. *65:* 29 (1935).
18   SPILSBURY, B.: Sudden death. Brit. Encyclopaedia med. Practice, vol. 3 (London 1937).
19   SUZMAN, M. and JOKL, E.: Sth afr. J. med. Sci. *1:* 206 (1936).
20   VISSCHER, M. B.: J. amer. med. Ass. *113:* 987 (1939).

Authors' address: University of Kentucky, *Lexington, KY 40506* (USA)

Medicine and Sport, vol. 5: Exercise and Cardiac Death, pp. 25-63
(Karger, Basel 1971)

Sudden Cardiac Death of Pilots in Flight

With Special Consideration of Syncope Due to Silent Ischemic Heart Disease and the Differential Diagnosis of Other Causes of Episodes of Incapacitation, Unconsciousness, Confusion and Amnesia in Flying Personnel

E. JOKL and J. T. McCLELLAN

'Silent' ischemic heart disease is the cause of unforeseen episodes of unconsciousness, confusion, amnesia and sudden death in pilots, by far the most important clinical problem in aviation medicine. Since the first discussion of this issue by SYMONDS and WILLIAMS [WILLIAMS, 1947] relevant information has become available through studies of a large number of cases of sudden unexpected non-traumatic death associated with exercise. These reports have shown that clinical manifestations of serious cardiac disease need not be in evidence prior to the onset of the terminal syncope, and that exercise capacity is not always a reliable prognostic criterion in cardiology. Ischemic heart disease causing sudden death in association with physical exertion in seemingly healthy subjects does not always develop silently. One must therefore distinguish those cases whose history is characterized by the appearance of signs and symptoms, as well as by an impairment of exercise capacity from those in which these diagnostic indicators are conspicuously absent. Aviation medicine is very much concerned with the first of these two categories. To have focused attention upon this apparent paradox is one of the major contributions which clinical sports medicine has made to functional pathology. In an attempt to outline nature and scope of the issue, we shall refer not only to cardiac problems sensu strictiori, but also to other clinical conditions that can cause unheralded *episodic unconsciousness, confusion, amnesia, syncope* and *death* during flight.

Fatal attack of angina pectoris in military pilot: In 1937 BENSON reported the history of a military pilot, age 35, who suffered his initial and fatal attack of angina pectoris while flying. No physical defects of note had been found at previous medical examinations. At the time of the anginal attack, this officer was the only pilot in the plane which carried several passengers.

Despite severe precordial pain, he flew for 20 min. to his destination and landed his plane without mishap. He died within 1 hour. Autopsy revealed a hypertrophied heart (411 G), advanced coronary arteriosclerosis and myocardial degeneration with fibrotic changes of the auricular-ventricular bundle. Had the pilot's death occurred in the air with a resultant crash, the conjectures as to the cause of the accident would have been unlimited.

Myocardial infarction in 34-year-old aviator. In 1940 GRAYBIEL and McFARLAND described a case of myocardial infarction in a 34-year-old aviator who had no complaints but was concerned because he had been told after a recent electrocardiographic examination that 'something was wrong with his heart.' He had taught in a flying school for a number of years and subsequently worked as a transport pilot. During World War II, he flew nonpressurized planes at altitudes of 18,000 feet; on one occasion he was forced down by hostile planes and landed in a small river. After providing life belts for the passengers, there was none left for himself. This circumstance saved his life, because he was able to dive under water to avoid machine gun bullets. When he reached safety, he was exhausted but recovered quickly. He had never complained of chest pains, dyspnoea, or palpitations. His pulse rate was 60/min, blood pressure 106/66 mm Hg. T waves were deeply inverted in Standard Leads I and II. From these findings a diagnosis was made of coronary heart disease and healed myocardial infarction without definite symptoms of coronary insufficiency.

In 1967, the US Civil Aeronautics Board reported 37 accidents in aviation due to incapacitation from cardiovascular disease, including the following 2 case accounts.

Case 1. 48-year-old private pilot was seen to be unconscious shortly after takeoff from the airport at Compton, California. The airplane continued a descending turn and crashed in a parking lot. *Post-mortem* examination revealed occlusion of both the left anterior descending and right coronary arteries with recent hemorrhage into the coronary lumen. Evidence of old myocardial infarctions was present. The cause of the accident was determined to be 'acute myocardial insufficiency due to 'severe calcific coronary atherosclerosis'.

Case 2. A 50-year-old private pilot was flying at night with his wife near Dallas, Texas. The pilot suddenly slumped over unconscious. His wife managed to crash-land the air-plane and survived. The *post-mortem* examination revealed that the pilot had marked atherosclerosis of the left coronary artery with 80-90% occlusion for a distance of 5 cm. The right coronary artery was similarly involved. Evidence (scarring of the myocardium) of a previous infarction was found.

Two years earlier the pilot had sustained a myocardial infarction and had 'recovered without difficulty.'

The following detailed case report was published by REIGHARD and
MOHLER [1967].

A Lockheed Electra crashed 1.5 miles north-east of the Ardmore, Oklahoma, Airport
at 8:30 p.m. on April 22, 1966. Of the 93 passengers and 5 crew members aboard, 18
passengers survived the initial crash. Three of these 18 died a little later due to the injuries.
The impact and subsequent fire destroyed the aircraft.

The flight crew had reported for duty at 0430 local time on the morning of April 22.
They were scheduled to fly from Ardmore to Lawton, Oklahoma, for a military charter
to McChord Air Force Base, Washington. From there they planned to fly to Monterey,
California, for a military charter flight to Columbus, Georgia. A crew change and refueling
stop was scheduled for Ardmore, Oklahoma, during this latter flight.

The pilot was 59 years old with 16,000 h total flight time and 1,200 h in Lockheed
Electra aircraft. He held a current Airline Transport Pilot certificate and his last first-class
medical certificate was issued February 22, 1966, just 2 months before the accident.

During the hours preceding the accident, the weather conditions at Ardmore were
very close to instrument approach minimums for the airport and the crew was aware of
this fact early in the flight. At the time of the accident the ceiling and visibility at the airport were officially reported above approved circling minimums. At the accident site,
the ceiling could have been on the order of 100 to 200 ft with 1¼-1½ mile visibility in
light rain showers and fog.

The aircraft was cleared to the Ardmore airport to cruise at 5,000 feet and the pilot
elected to make an ADF approach to runway 8 and at 2026 local time the pilot reported
he was inbound and over the radio beacon. According to witnesses the aircraft passed
approximately 1 mile north of the beacon and turned to the northeast establishing a track
of approximately 71° magnetic. The track from the beacon to the airport placed the aircraft about 1¾-2 miles north of runway 8 in an east-northeasterly direction. The altitude
of the plane varied from 1,200 to 963 ft msl during the last 75 sec. Unfortunately the flight
recorder aboard the aircraft was not functioning properly at the time of the accident.

The FAA flight service specialist at Ardmore had the aircraft in sight when it was
approximately 2 miles northwest of the airport when the crew requested a change of lights
from runway 8 to runway 12. The flight should not have descended below 1,362 ft msl
unless the aircraft was clear of the clouds. It was determined that the aircraft did descend
to approximately 1,160 ft at which altitude it was observed north of the airport and it
crashed at 963 ft msl.

After the initial impact the aircraft came to rest in approximately 750 ft. Most of
the wreckage was consumed by fire after the aircraft came to a stop. Most of the passenger
seats separated from the aircraft and tumbled out onto the ground during the last 150 ft
of aircraft travel.

Amidst the wreckage was found a partially burned role of glucose 'Tes-Tape' which
is normally used to test for the presence of sugar in the urine. Also found in the wreckage
were 2 types of pills and a small empty prescription bottle labeled with the pilot's name.
One of the pills was identified as nitroglycerin, and the other was determined to be
Tolbutamide.

A *post-mortem* examination performed on the pilot revealed the presence of severe
coronary atherosclerosis. There was a fracture of the right ulna, a fracture of the left

lateral epicondyle, and a fracture of the left index and ring fingers. Examination of the copilot revealed a comminuted fracture of the right humerus, a comminuted fracture of the right ulna and radius; fractures of the metacarpal head of the thumb of the right hand; a compound comminuted fracture of the left thumb; and a fracture dislocation through the medial epicondyle. An aviation pathologist testified that the injuries to the first officer's hand and arms indicated that his hands could have been on the controls of the aircraft at the time of the accident. Such injuries were not found on the captain's hands. Prior to the time of the accident the copilot had been handling the radio transmissions and it had been presumed that the captain had been handling the controls.

An investigation was accomplished into the pilot's past medical history. His medical records revealed that the first indications of coronary artery disease existed as early as 1947. From that time until 1950 he made many visits to his personal physician, the records of which presented increasing evidence, from a historical standpoint, of major heart disease. From 1950 until 1963 there was no record of any complaints about the patient's heart, but from 1963 until his last visit in April 11, 1966, there was an indication that the patient was having symptoms characterized by chest pain which radiated down the left arm. During this period the captain received prescriptions for various medications including aminophylline, nitroglycerin, and peritrate. Subsequent to 1963, peritrate was taken 4 times daily and the prescription had been refilled 26 times. The records also revealed that the captain had been taking Orinase, $1\frac{1}{2}$ tablet a day since October 1962, for the control of diabetes mellitus.

During these periods of treatment the captain was taking semi-annual FAA Class 1 flight physicals, which also included ECGs. He obtained these examinations from a designated Aviation Medical Examiner, from whom the pilot withheld details of treatment by his personal physician. A review of the applications for medical certificates completed by the captain showed that he denied having had either heart disease or diabetes. He also had denied having consulted a physician or being under medication.

It was the conclusion of the Civil Aeronautics Board that after missing the approach to runway 8, the captain flew north of the airport for an approach and landing on another runway. While attempting a right turn the captain experienced coronary insufficiency and became incapable of controlling the aircraft. This caused the aircraft to descend below the minimum altitude before the first officer could effectively recover control of the aircraft prior to the impact. Both the captain and first officer had been aloft approximately 11 h during 16 h duty time, and the CAB felt that fatigue from 16 h duty time contributed to the captain's susceptibility to incapacitation.

The CAB determined the probable cause of the accident to be incapacitation, due to coronary insufficiency, of the pilot-in-command at a critical point during a visual circling approach being conducted under instrument flight conditions.

In 1968 JOKL and McCLELLAN published a report of the sudden death in flight of a 50-year-old pilot of a passenger plane and 'Director of Safety' of the Airline for which he flew. He had over 700 flying hours to his credit over a period of 14 years and was thought to be in perfect health. A recent physical examination had yielded 'no positive findings.' He had been on a vacation to Florida during which he freely participated in recreational activities. On the day of his death, he played 18 holes of golf, walking the entire course before piloting a plane carrying 4 passengers from Vero Beach, Florida, northward. While flying at an altitude of 5,500 ft over Kentucky, he complained of shortness of breath and asked that the windows of the plane be opened. A few minutes later he slumped over dead. There was no co-pilot in the cockpit. One of the passengers came to the rescue and landed the plane at the Blue Grass Airport in Kentucky.

A *post-mortem* examination was performed at St. Joseph's Hospital in Lexington, Kentucky. The significant findings relate to heart and lungs.

The heart weighed 500 g. Right atrium and ventricle showed no abnormalities; the foramen ovale was closed; left atrium and left ventricle were enlarged. An *aneurysmatic* bulge was noted near the apex. Mitral and aortic valves were slightly thickened. The coronary ostia originated at the usual sites and were patent. The *left* branch of the coronary artery was *occluded* in two places by thrombi, the one red brown and without signs of organization, the other organized. The *circumflex* artery was *totally obstructed* by atheromatous plaques. The *right* coronary artery was blocked over a distance of half an inch by a *fresh massive hemorrhage* into an organized atheromatous plaque. The *myocardium* of the left ventricle near the apex showed reddish discoloration suggestive of *infarction*. Scattered *fibrous scars* measuring up to 1 cm in diameter were noted in septum and wall of the left ventricle (fig. 1-4). The lungs were heavy, boggy, and wet, exuding pink, frothy material from cut surfaces. Histological examination of pulmonary tissue revealed numerous macrophages laden with hemosiderin. There were no acute inflammatory infiltrates.

Six months prior to the fatal collapse, the deceased had last been seen by a physician, in connection with his statutory annual 'Application for Airman Medical Certificate'. The printed sheet prescribed for the recording of medical history contained only 2 questions pertaining to heart and blood vessels, namely 'Have you ever had or have you now heart trouble?', and 'Do you have high or low blood pressure?' The answers to both were negative. The examining physician entered into the record that 'Heart (thrust, size, rhythm, sounds)' and 'The Vascular System' were 'normal': that blood pressure was 110/74 mm Hg; pulse rate at rest 74/min; 'after exercise' 108/min; 2 min after exercise' 72/min. No other data concerning the cardiovascular system are contained in the official examination form FAA-1004 (6–60).

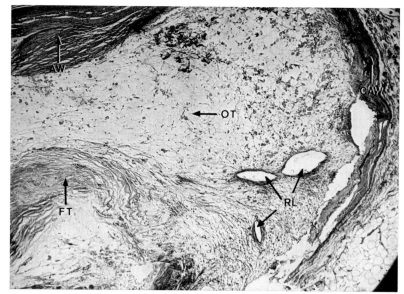

Fig. 1. Left anterior descending coronary artery (x 10). AW=Arterial Wall (thickened intima); FT=Fibrous Tissue; CAW=Calcified Arterial Wall; OT=Organized Thrombus; RL=Recanalized Lumina.

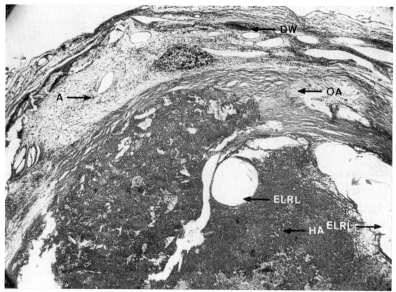

Fig. 2. Right coronary artery (x 10). A=Atheroma; DW=Degenerated Wall; OA=Organized Atheroma; HA=Hemorrhage in Atheroma; ELRL=Endothelial Lined Recanalized Lumina.

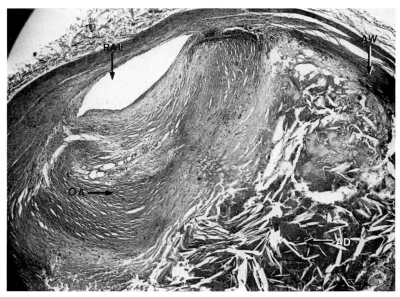

Fig. 3. Circumflex coronary artery (x 10). RAL=Remaining Arterial Lumen; AW =Artery Wall; OA=Organized Atheroma; AD=Atheromatous Deposit with Cholesterol Clefts.

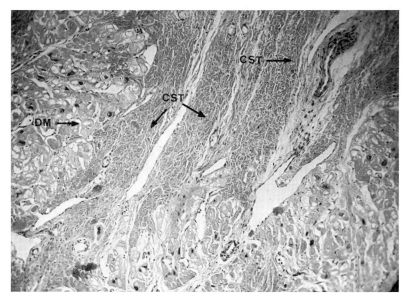

Fig. 4. Interventricular septum (x 10). CST=Collagenous Scar Tissue (old infarction); DM=Degenerating Myocardium.

Summarizing their findings, JOKL and MCCLELLAN wrote that the autopsy revealed advanced atheromatous coronary artery disease with cardiac hypertrophy and myocardial degeneration. The natural history of the pathological process must have extended over several years. Extensive myocardial infarctions involved the apical portion of the left ventricle and the interventricular septum. Organized thrombi occluded portions of the main stem of the left coronary artery and its circumflex branch.

Effect of altitude on coronary heart disease. In 1941 GRAYBIEL drew attention to the fact that patients with manifest coronary heart disease and angina pectoris may tolerate reduced oxygen tension without developing pain. He subjected 4 such patients to a simulated altitude of 14,500 ft for periods as long as 45 min. None of them developed pain.

The case of a middle-aged man who died following coronary occlusion and in whom autopsy showed marked coronary atherosclerosis and myocardial infarction was particularly striking. Less than 3 years before his death, he had been a member of a high altitude expedition to Chile, during which he experienced no more difficulty than other members of the party at elevations up to 20,000 ft. After his return, he acted both as subject and investigator for numerous experiments of 3- to 5-h duration at simulated altitudes of 15,000 to 17,000 ft. Toward the end of a test in which the inhaled oxygen concentration was 10.5%, he performed a standing run which carried him near to collapse.

Autopsy studies of coronary arteries of 222 military aviators. In 1959 GLANTZ and STEMBRIDGE examined sections of heart and coronary arteries of 222 military aviators who had died in air crashes. The age range of the group was 19 to 43; 64% were between 20 and 30, paralleling the overall age distribution in the US Air Force. In 70% of the cases 'some degree of coronary artery atherosclerosis was demonstrable'; in 21% there was atherosclerosis of 'moderate to marked degree'. In several instances the lumen of the coronary artery or one of its branches was diminished by more than three-quarters.

Incidence of coronary artery disease in young adults. In 1960 RIGAL *et al.* published a report which contained an evaluation of the incidence of coronary artery disease in young people based upon autopsy records of 206 military flying and 165 non-flying personnel, all of whom had met with accidental death. Samples were matched so as to render a comparison with the autopsy findings reported by GLANTZ and STEMBRIDGE [1959] possible. The results of these two studies were in close agreement; they also confirmed earlier observations of ENOS, HOLMES and BEYER [1953] who found gross evidence of coronary arterial sclerosis in 77.3% of autopsies performed on 300 US soldiers killed in action in Korea. GLANTZ and STEMBRIDGE [1959] and RIGAL et al. [1960] found but little sclerosis in the aorta, the renal arcuate arteries, the small arteries of the periadrenal fat, and the pancreatic arteries. They concluded that in young men free of clinical evidence of ischemic heart disease, coronary atherosclerosis develops at a more rapid rate than in arteries of other organs.

Cardiovascular system of aging pilots. SCHREUDER and CONSTANTINO [1960] published an analysis of the records of 150 active pilots over 40 years of age (15 of them between 51 and 60). Five (3%) exhibited arterial hypertension; 13 (9%) were overweight; 2 (1%) had border line cardiac hypertrophy; 11 (7%) exhibited minor electrocardiographic changes. All of them were entirely without symptoms. So were 20 among 186 applicants for the position of co-pilots who were rejected because of the discovery during the screening examination of chronic cardiovascular defects.[1]

Relevance of post-mortem findings of coronary artery disease in the evaluation of unexplained aircraft accidents. Summarizing the evidence detailed in the Proceedings of the 1959 'Symposium on Cardiology in Aviation', LAMB et al. [1960] wrote that caution must be employed in implicating coronary artery disease as a causative factor in otherwise unexplained aircraft accidents. 'A finding of narrowing of the lumen of the coronary arteries must be weighed in the light of information of mechanical factors pertaining to the accident.' Referring to the Armed Forces Institute of Pathology's autopsy records obtained from flying personnel killed in accidents, TOWNSEND [1964] confirmed the earlier observation that silent coronary artery disease in young people is less likely to be accompanied by degenerative arterial changes in other parts of the body than it is in middle-aged or older groups.

Electrocardiographic studies of flying personnel. In electrocardiographic studies of 67,375 asymptomatic cases of flying personnel, 2,519 abnormalities were discovered by LAMB et al. [1960]. There was a significant

---

1   See appendix 1.

increase with age of the incidence of non-specific T-wave changes, ventricular ectopic beats, right bundle branch block, and myocardial infarction. Premature ventricular contractions were noted in 419 instances. Of these, 22 were extrasystoles, one multifocal. There was a twofold rise in the incidence of premature ventricular contractions in the 40–44 age group, as compared with younger men, and a threefold rise in those above 45 years of age. A Wolff-Parkinson-White syndrome was observed in 109 cases. There were 13 cases of complete left bundle branch block and 106 cases of complete right bundle branch block.

Prognostic significance of abnormal T wave in fighter command-pilot. In 1960 MANNING reported the medical history of a 27-year-old pilot in whom a routine electrocardiographic examination had revealed 'an abnormal T wave'. This man was in apparent good health and continued to serve as a fighter command-pilot engaged in operational flights. One year after the T-wave changes were discovered, he died suddenly as he approached his aircraft for a take-off. The cause of death was reported as coronary thrombosis. MANNING mentions that other examples have occurred in which the ECG indicated a cardiac disorder not recognized clinically among 17,000 fit, healthy young men 18 to 24 years of age, examined at the Institute of Aviation Medicine of the Royal Canadian Air Force.

Comparison of rates of incidence of coronary artery disease in RAF and USAF. In 1962 MASON reported a 34.4% incidence of coronary artery disease in the Royal Air Force aircrew population, a figure somewhat below that observed in the USAF. On the whole, both investigations established that coronary artery disease is widespread in all age groups among British as well as U.S. airmen; and that incidence and severity of the disease increase with age.

Post-mortem findings in aircraft accident victims who had military flight status. In 1963 CATHERMAN et al. reviewed *post-mortem* findings in 463 aircraft accident victims who had military flight status. Coronary atherosclerosis was found in 76% of the cases. In the age group 20 to 43, significant coronary involvement was present in 38%. In 80% of the aircraft accidents, there was sufficient evidence of cause other than coronary artery disease. In a series of 96 cardiac autopsies, the authors found a significant degree of coronary artery atherosclerosis and myocardial fibrosis in 15% of the cases.

1965 Bethesda Conference on 'Standards of Physical Fitness of Aircrew'.
On November 6 and 7, 1965, a conference was held on 'Standards of
Physical Fitness of Aircrew' in Bethesda, Maryland. The proceedings
emphasized that the age of pilots is steadily advancing as they are now
allowed to maintain their commercial licenses until the age of 60 years.
Thus, there is a greater tendency to atherosclerosis with resulting cerebral
and myocardial catastrophic events. Reports indicate that several commercial air disasters have been caused by such catastrophic vascular events
during landing or take-off when the co-pilot did not have time to take
over the controls.

Appended to the Conference Report was a paper by WEBSTER and
HOFFMAN [1966] which surveys the literature on coronary disease in a
young aircraft population. The paper notes the striking absence of cases
of thrombosis and fatal infarction in the cases reviewed.

Heart disease and flying status. In 1967 COOPER reported the case of
a 31-year-old US Air Force pilot who was grounded when an ECG taken
on Nov. 25, 1964, revealed changes indicative of myocardial ischemia.

ST-segments in leads II and a Vf were depressed; T waves in lead III inverted.
An ECG recorded during a routine examination a year earlier (on Nov. 27, 1963) had been
normal.

The ECG was repeated on Nov. 30, 1964. Inversion of the T waves in lead II, III and
a Vf was now even more distinct. A history of epigastric discomfort and of episodes of
'indigestion' was elicited. The patient's father had died suddenly at age 57, presumably of a
heart attack. A harsh, early systolic sound, probably extracardiac, was heard along the
lower left sternal border, increasing with expiration and decreasing with inspiration.
ECGs recorded on December 1, 1964, and on December 2, 1964, showed persistence of
the T-wave anomalies.

On December 17, 1964, the patient developed bronchopneumonia. No etiological
agent could be identified. Response to treatment was good and the ECG changes improved
during the acute illness. A chest X-ray obtained on November 25, 1964, was reviewed and
interpreted as normal. So were several subsequent roentgenograms taken during 'the
presence of maximum ECG abnormality'.

ECG tracings taken on January 7, 1965, at rest as well as following 'stress procedures', including tilting and exercise, showed no abnormalities.

Because of the findings and the possibility of recurrent ischemic episodes, the patient
could not be recommended for return to unrestricted flying status and was grounded perma-
nently. Final diagnoses were myocardial infarction and probable coronary artery disease.

At this stage the patient initiated a physical training program. He practised regularly, at times twice daily, during the ensuing 18 months. At the end of this period he was
capable of running 25 miles in 3 h. Coronary angiography showed no evidence of anatomic
atherosclerotic disease. The cardiac arteries were conspicuously large.

These findings as well as views expressed by the Conference on 'Standards of Physical Fitness of Conference on Aircrew' to the effect that civilian pilots with a history of myocardial infarction may be returned to flying duties if adequately rehabilitated induced the medical authorities to rescind their earlier decision. The patient was given a waiver for an 'abnormal ECG' and reinstated to full flying duties.

Prognostic value of exercise capacity in the assessment of coronary risk after myocardial infarction. We do not agree that high physical performance standards justify reinstatement of pilots to flying duties after myocardial infarction. Indeed little or no correlation exists between exercise capacity and probability of sudden death occurring in subjects with ischemic heart disease. One of the most significant results obtained in our long-term study of sudden cardiac deaths in athletes is that the disease often remains 'silent' and renders unrestricted participation in physical activities possible. We do not know why subjects in whom autopsy first revealed the presence of advanced coronary and myocardial disease collapsed and died when they did. The same question is also unanswerable when sudden fatal cardiac collapse occurs in persons who prior to their death did present signs and symptoms of coronary heart disease and whose exercise capacity was critically reduced. We simply do not know the ultimate causes of terminal attacks of ventricular fibrillation or cardiac stand-still. The adaptations that determine exercise capacity are of a physiological nature. In 1897 WILLIAM H. WELCH, master pupil of JULIUS COHNHEIM, presented his classical paper entitled 'Adaptations in Pathological Processes', in which he showed that adaptations in *pathological* processes follow patterns of their own that differ categorically from those which occur in *physiological situations*. To draw conclusions from the appropriateness of the latter as to their *clinical* effectiveness is definitely not permissible.[2]

Routine medical examination of pilots. In 1967 LANE reviewed the results of medical examinations of Australian airline pilots during the period 1953–1965, comprising populations of 900 in 1953 and of 1400 in 1965. Between 1953 and 1965 the age distribution of the men changed because the sample included many pilots who had been trained in World

2   For a detailed description and discussion of the Cohnheim-Welch theory, see JOKL, *Clinical Physiology of Physical Fitness and Rehabilitation* (Thomas, 1958).

War II. 52 pilots were disqualified for medical reasons. Of these, 75% had reported health problems during the currency of their license. The medical status of the 13 others came to light at regular physical examinations, i.e., the men did not know or, if they did, had failed to reveal the presence of illness. In 7 cases the physical deficiencies diagnosed at the examination were not regarded sufficient to justify cancellation of the license. The subjects — among them 2 senior commercial pilots — continued to be under medical surveillance and attended to their duties as pilots for periods ranging from 6 months to 15 years. In 2 men the results of routine electro-cardiographic examinations led to disqualification.

LANE pointed out that 'the ECG is not routinely required at each medical examination but at intervals, depending upon age, which may be as long as 10 years decreasing to 1 year at minimum. ECGs are required, as a routine, at the first airline transport pilot examination, at age 30, 35, 40, 2 yearly to 50, then annually.'

The 5 residual cases were as follows: The first concerned a pilot in whom the diagnosis 'anxiety state' was made. This man ceased flying voluntarily and was classified as 'failing to meet medical standards'. His license was cancelled. Another pilot who at the time of the regular medical examination had no complaints of ill health was found to have an enlarged spleen. A blood examination led to a diagnosis of chronic myeloid leukemia. Renewal of his license was refused. He was reinstated 6 months later, being allowed to fly as co-pilot. 14 months after the original diagnosis, he died following an acute phase of his condition. LANE believes that in cases of this kind, 'sudden incapacity does not seem likely'. The third case is that of a 47-year-old airline pilot who had a fainting attack just prior to his regular physical check-up. There was a history of chest pain over a period of 9 months during which he had passed a routine medical examination. On the basis of his information, a full cardiovascular investigation was carried out and his license revoked. It is noteworthy that the disease had not been identified earlier though he had brought his fainting attack to the attention of his family doctor.

The fourth history relates to an airline pilot, age 27, who had consulted his doctor for recurrent furuncles, was found to have lost weight and to exhibit glycosuria. A glucose tolerance test established the diagnosis of diabetes [CATLETT and KIDERA, 1965; WILLIAMS; 1966].

The last case concerned a senior commercial pilot, age 49, who was noted by the medical examiner to have a swollen cheek but received permission to continue flying pending further tests. His condition was eventually found to be a cancer of the maxillary antrum. He received X-ray treatment which led to a marked impairment of the vision of one eye. He therefore was disqualified and died some 8 months later.

'*Aviator's cancer*'. Under this heading, ANDREWS and MICHAELS [1968] reported similar cases from Canada, which suggested that the frequent barometric pressure changes experienced by bush pilots may have played a part in the causation of the malignancies. We quote without comment:

'The bush pilots of Canada have led an adventurous, exacting, and lonely life. The difficulties of high-altitude navigation, the uncertainties of radio communication, and the severities of the sub-Arctic winter combine in formidable opposition to the free-lance aviators, upon whom so many small outposts depend. Though the stages they fly are usually short, they must be prepared to put down in almost any sort of terrain, on wheels, floats, or skis: and, if forced down by the weather, they may have to stay where they are, living as best they can, for a week or more, until the persistent Arctic fog lifts. But such are the difficulties of surface movement that the aeroplane, in face of all the risks, is the best, sometimes the only, means of transport and communication between scattered communities. So the bush pilots have been in great demand. During their careers they spend many thousands of hours in the air mainly in short trips in unpressurised aircraft: each climb and descent exposes the pilot to barometric pressure change, with consequent ventilation of the middle ear: and during the descent there is generally need for voluntary effort, the Valsalva manoeuvre, to equilibrate the pressure. In some way these continual movements of air along the Eustachian tubes may eventually lead to changes in the epithelium.

There are, of course, other groups of airmen all over the world, who work under similar conditions of barometric change, at as great or even greater intensity — crop-duster, air taxi, and helicopter pilots, for example. It remains to be seen whether tumours of the nasopharynx arise more often in these than in other occupations. But even if there is no such experience elsewhere, there remains the possibility that pressure change may still be a cause — when combined with some other factor peculiar to the country. There may, for example, be a climatic peculiarity: the very cold, dry air of the Canadian winter can be painful to breathe even at ground level. Perhaps a combination of insults may induce the neoplastic change: tiny spicules of ice in movement may be no less destructive than tiny spicules of wood.' [3]

'Relatively sudden death' in airline pilots. LANE [1967] reports on 11 'relatively sudden deaths' in airline pilots. Of these, 2 were due to cerebral tumor, 2 to rupture of a congenital intracranial aneurysm, and 4 to cardio-vascular disease. In 7 of them the pathological condition had not been detected or suspected at the preceding regular medical examination. Between January 1960 and June 1965, there were 16 deaths of airline pilots during the currency of their licenses. Among them was a pilot, aged 40, who died in a hospital undiagnosed with an acute illness, whose autopsy showed rupture of a large abscess of the liver due to a chronic amoebic infection. He had passed his regular medical examination by a

3   See appendix 2.

specialist physician 2 days before the onset of his illness and 15 days before his death. Finally, there is the case of a flight captain, aged 44, whose aircraft crashed for no obvious reason on approach to landing. *Post-mortem* examination disclosed isolated myocarditis as probable cause of the accident. The deceased had had a medical examination 3 months earlier during which no cardiac anomalies were detected.

Cardiological criteria for evaluation of flying status. The data at hand leave no doubt that among healthy young US flyers the incidence of moderate or marked atherosclerosis of the coronary arteries is the same as in non-flying military personnel. The diagnostic criteria applied in the evaluation of the circulatory system of older pilots do not differ from those applied to younger men. This is so notwithstanding the fact mentioned earlier that *post-mortem* evidence obtained from aircrew populations and athletes alike indicates a relation between presence and severity of coronary heart disease, and increasing age. From the results of his autopsy studies of accidentally killed Royal Air Force flying personnel, MASON [1962] concluded that the increase in severity of coronary atherosclerosis in relation to the number of hours flown is significant only because it reflects advancing age. Altogether the relationship between coronary heart disease and age of pilots represents only a statistically demonstrable trend. SCHREUDER and CONSTANTINO [1960] describe the case of a 36-year-old pilot whose application to be reinstated after being off flight duty for 5 weeks because of 'an acute non-specific pericarditis' was rejected when the medical examination revealed evidence of a recent anteroseptal infarction. Four years later, this man died from acute coronary occlusion. The question has been asked whether the cumulative stress of flying represents a pathogenetic factor in the development of coronary heart disease. There is no evidence to support such a hypothesis.

The role of exercise in the elicitation of sudden fatal collapse. The pilot whose fatal collapse in flight is reported on p. 32 had played 18 holes of golf immediately prior to his death. There are many similar observations of persons who had been exercising or even participating in athletic contest shortly before they dropped dead. One therefore may ask whether exercise predisposes to attacks of ventricular fibrillation or cardiac standstill in subjects with silent or clinically manifest atherosclerotic coronary heart disease.[4] The evidence at hand is inconclusive. Our own clinical and autopsy

4   See appendix 3.

data on sudden cardiac death associated with exercise suggest that occasionally such cause-and-effect sequences cannot be ruled out, though pathogenetic factors, other than those referred to earlier, were involved in most cases which seemed to comply with the prerequisites for such a hypothesis.[5]

Contributing causative factors. In a 16-year-old high school student who died while playing basketball, we found *post-mortem* a congenital anomaly of the left coronary artery. The structural defect had not prevented the boy from participating in vigorous sport activities over many years. We also noted at autopsy multiple bronchiolar obstructions secondary to numerous small mucous plugs due to a diffuse widespread bilateral inflammatory process presumably of viral origin.

The autopsy of a 10-year-old boy, who died during a boxing fight, showed a fresh hemorrhage into an atheromatous and calcified plaque. The latter formed part of an organized thrombus that completely obstructed the left coronary artery. The hemorrhage had presumably been caused by several blunt traumata to the chest during the pugilistic encounter [JOKL and GREENSTEIN, 1944].

DENNEY and READ [1965] reported the 'scuba diving death' of a 38-year-old swimmer whose autopsy revealed a freshly formed thrombus in the descending coronary artery, probably caused as a result of the abnormal respiratory pressure and pulmonary oxygenation patterns during the dive. PUGH [1966], and MONGE and MONGE [1966] have presented evidence to the effect that thermoregulatory adjustments necessitated by environmental temperature extremes, if added to adaptive requirements of physical exercise under conditions of reduced atmospheric pressure, can overtax the resources of the autonomic system and cause death.

Genetic determinants of onset of fatal collapse in association with strenuous physical exertion. There are on record observations of sudden non-traumatic death associated with physical exertion in identical twins which have a bearing on the question of the endogenous as against extraneous determinants of the time of onset of fatal collapses whose primary causes could be identified at autopsy. In 1942 CLUVER and JOKL analyzed the death of a 32-year-old international rugby football player who collapsed and died immediately after a strenuous game.

5   See appendix 4.

The case created a sensation since the deceased had been known as 'The Iron Man of Rugby'. *Post-mortem* examination revealed general hypertrophy of the heart which weighed 482 g. The hypertrophy was most apparent in the left ventricle which measured 2.7 cm in thickness. All cavities of the heart were dilated. Numerous fibrotic patches were irregularly distributed throughout the wall of the left ventricle. There was widespread atheromatosis, more particularly in the coronary artery. The left branch of the coronary artery was markedly narrowed at 3 places. The aorta was extraordinarily soft and thin. The descending portion of the vessel measured little over $\frac{1}{2}$ in in diameter which is less than the normal size. Excess lymphoid tissue was found in the spleen and in the thymus gland which weighed 26 g (normal weight 15 g) and which contained active Hassal's bodies. The left kidney was small (62 g) and was the seat of advanced hydronephrosis. The parenchyma was stretched and thinned and the pelvis was much dilated. The left ureter was sharply kinked about 1 in above the bladder. The right kidney was hypertrophied (330 g). Genital organs were small.

The deceased had an identical twin brother who a few months earlier had also died during exertion (swimming).

O'BRIEN [1942] has reported a somewhat similar pattern with identical twins.

One twin, a previously healthy adult, age 26, while playing tennis complained of severe headache and became subsequently unconscious. He died the following morning. The diagnosis of subarachnoid hemorrhage was made, but no autopsy was carried out. Soon afterwards the deceased's identical twin brother who had been employed on a farm pulling sugar beets was found dead in an empty house. *Post-mortem* examination revealed a hemorrhagic cyst in the middle of the right hemisphere beneath the Rolandic area about 4 cm in diameter, with a pigmented wall. Near the origin of the left middle cerebral artery was a thrombosed aneurysm about 1 cm in diameter. Adhesions and pigmentation of the surrounding tissues pointed to leakage. The brain was congested and oedematous and covered with thick pus over the base.

'Terminal trigger mechanisms'. The presence of coronary disease as such does not necessarily explain fatal syncope even though anginal attacks during flight are known to affect the ability of flying personnel to control the aircraft. Nor is evidence of recent morphological changes invariably encountered at autopsies of sujects who died suddenly from coronary atherosclerosis. Fresh thrombi or peri-atheromatous hemorrhages have been found at times but we have equally often failed to discover sequelae of acute vascular or perivascular disturbance. Such observations suggest that the onset of terminal phases of at least some of the fatal collapses can be of functional origin, whatever this term may imply. The fact that collapses which at first seem to herald death may turn out not to be terminal and to reverse spontaneously is in agreement with such a theory. HELLERSTEIN has presented a case of spontaneous reversion of cardiac asystole lasting 100 sec. It occurred after exercise in a man with hypercholesteremia, xanthomatosis, aortic stenosis, and a history of myocardial infarction, who was reportedly alive 5 years

following the electrocardiographically verified long episode of ventricular standstill.

BERNARD LOWEN and WILLIAM RUBERMAN have recently discussed the problem of identifying 'populations at risk from sudden death due to coronary atherosclerotic heart disease'. ('The Concept of Precoronary Care,' Modern Concepts of Cardiovascular Disease, May, 1970). A distinction must be made, they say, between three groups: (1) patients with acute cardiac infarction, (2) patients with coronary atherosclerotic heart disease and symptoms but without evidence of infarction, and (3) subjects dying suddenly without overt prodromes.

While sudden death accounts for the major fraction of coronary mortality, the group of athletes or pilots whose deaths were studied by us represent a category of their own in that they had failed to show overt clinical prodromes prior to the terminal collapse. They also had been able to perform physically *usque ad finem*. The question arises whether in such persons the cardiac affliction can be discovered 'in good time', e.g. during the annual medical examination of pilots. This is possible but may be difficult. For example, a normal ECG is compatible with the presence of acute myocardial infarction. Contrariwise during routine examinations of seemingly healthy athletes ECG have been recorded that would have to be considered indicative of acute myocardial infarction if encountered in patients seen in clinical practice.

The most threatened among the heterogenous population groups at risk from sudden death are mostly identifiable through documentation of multiple premature ventricular beats (VPB). Frequencies of 10/1000 cycles or more signify a tenfold greater risk of cardiac death among actively employed men of 55 and older. VPB are of no clinical significance if they occur in young and vigorous persons, a fact first noted by JOKL 40 years ago (Med. Klinik, Nr. 32, 1933). To discover older individuals afflicted with CAHD and who have PVB it is necessary to monitor them electrocardiographically over long periods, but in 'Precoronary Care Areas' equipped with on-line data reduction analogue or digital instrumentation.

Acute terminal episodes in subjects afflicted with atherosclerotic coronary heart disease are invariably superimposed on chronic progressive pathological changes. The distinction between long term and transient coronary risk factors is of fundamental importance.

Electrical instability of the heart is the best known diagnostic parameter to be searched for in subjects of the kind under discussion, moreover ventricular fibrillation and cardiac standstill are ubiquitous mediators of sudden unexpected cardiac death in athletes and flying personnel. Likewise, acute fatal subendothelial hemorrhages and fresh intravascular thrombi are invariably heralded.

Episodes of unconsciousness, confusion and amnesia while flying. A variety of cardiac as well as extracardiac events are included among the terminal trigger mechanisms that may initiate sudden death in athletes or pilots. We know much more about 'primary pathological causes' of sudden cardiac death than about the modalities of elicitation of the fatal attacks. More than 20 years ago, WILLIAMS [1947] emphasized a problem of crucial importance to aviation medicine, namely that of 'Episodes of unconsciousness, confusion, and amnesia while flying': 'Attention has too often been directed to special conditions and to special investigations, and away from a consideration of the whole patient in relation to his total physical and psychological environment.'

ROOK [1947] categorized the symptomatology of disturbances of consciousness in previously fit men into amnesia, confusion, and transient giddiness or dizziness with tremitus to complete loss of consciousness, with or without convulsion. He distinguished 3 mechanisms leading to attacks: disturbances on the highest cortical levels, hypersensitivity of lower levels of the central nervous system causing explosive discharges or pathological inhibition, and disturbances of the blood supply to the brain. Emotion, ROOK [1947] wrote, may be 'the trigger that unloosens an epileptic fit or causes an attack of syncope'. He recalled GOWER's statement in 1907 that 'epilepsy and cardiovascular syncope appear to have a common meeting place in the brain'; that the line between fainting and fits cannot be sharply drawn; and that all symptoms or combinations of symptoms that occur in a grand mal attack can also result from cerebral anemia.[6]

Impairment of consciousness in RAF personnel during World War II. Of 500 cases of impairement of consciousness in apparently fit flying personnel of the Royal Air Force, 121 (24%) were considered 'primarily neurogenic', 154 (31%) 'primarily due to some cardiovascular cause', and 208 (42%) 'primarily emotional in origin'. The rest could not be classified. The incidence of syncopal unconsciousness in the Royal Air Force fell considerably towards the end of the war. ROOK [1947] ascribed this to 'the predominant part of psychological influences', and quoted a general's remark that 'men of a conquering army do not report sick'.

6   See appendix 5.

The incidence of *idiopathic epilepsy* among pilots and air crews in the war was between 1.1 and 1.3 $^o/_{oo}$. 121 of the 500 cases were 'primarily neurogenic'; 53, major idiopathic epilepsy; 6, 'doubtful major idiopathic epilepsy'; 10, 'minor idiopathic epilepsy'; 20, 'single convulsive attacks'; 5, cerebral neoplasm; 13, loss of consciousness after injury; 9, vertigo or aural origin; 5, miscellaneous.

Unsuspected neurological disease in aviation personnel. Two cases of 'Unsuspected Neurologic Disease in Aviation Personnel' were reported by SEIPEL and WENTZ.

One patient was a 53-year-old pilot who had several blackout spells due to temporal lobe convulsion disorder causing uncinate seizures. There had been episodes of blackout or fainting in childhood. At age 46, the patient had lost consciousness while piloting his plane solo. He was 'out' for about 30 min. When he regained consciousness, he was lying straight in the seat of the cockpit with his head resting in one corner of the seat. The plane continued to be air-born while the controles were unattended. The pilot eventually succeeded in regaining control and landing his aircraft. On the ground he remained in the cockpit for several minutes before feeling strong enough to get out of the cockpit. At this time he noted dryness of the mouth, drank a coke at the airport terminal, rested for 45 min, before resuming the flight. A physician whom he consulted, during the ensuing week told him that the episode must have been due to 'nerves and fatigue', but that is was 'all right' for him to continue flying. A psychiatrist said his symptoms were caused by 'business tension'. *Neither of the two doctors took steps to suspend the pilot's licence.*

Two years later, again while flying, the patient experienced a sensation of strange taste and odor and a feeling of tingling and itching. During the following years, similar attacks occurred frequently, while he flew, none of them at this stage of his illness accompanied by loss of consciousness.

During a glucose tolerance test, the electroencephalogram became dysrythmic. Numerous sharp waves and high voltage burts were recorded over the left temporal area, concommitant with a hypoglycemic episode.

A second case concerned a 34-year-old who was referred for neurological studies because of unexplained episodes of loss of consciousness while he flew as a co-pilot on a night mission. According to the pilot in charge of the plane, the patient was 'out' for a quarter of an hour. He slumped to the right side of the cockpit, striking his head with considerable force, injuring his nose.

The seizure occurred unheralded. There had been no known prior episodes of a similar kind. Sixteen years earlier he suffered a skull fracture in an automobile accident, which had rendered him unconscious for 24 h. During the ensuing years, he worked as a steeple jack without incident.

The neurological examination was unremarkable, except for a hearing defect on the left side and a 'minor memory deficit'. The pneumoencephalogram revealed an enlarged right ventricule due to unilateral atrophy of cortical and sub-cortical structures. The electroencephalogram showed evidence of diffuse dysrhythmia and asymmetry of amplitude with higher voltage activity on the left side evoked by hyperventilation. The recent grand mal seizure during the flight was considered due to a right cortical focal component, probably cerebral atrophy and scarring caused by the trauma 16 years ago. *Recertification was denied.*

Primary cardiovascular disease existed in most cases. Five cases had been thought to be due to hemorrhage, 25 due to infection, 7 due to pain, 7 due to 'black-out', 10 due to 'organic heart disease', 18 due to fatigue, 15 due to heat, 19 due to hypotension, 31 due to 'cardiovascular failure', and 17 miscellaneous. One case resulted from rupture of the splenic artery in an airman who had extricated himself from the rear turret, a feat of difficulty necessitating forced hypertension of the spine.

Among the 25 cases in which *infection* was considered to be the cause of syncope were 3 cases of active pulmonary tuberculosis, 3 of latent malaria, 3 of tonsillitis, 4 of upper respiratory tract infection, 2 of sinusitis and 2 with unexplained fever. Other infections included jaundice, kalaazar and bacilluria.

In 10 instances impairment of consciousness was considered 'due to heart lesions'. In 4 cases there was a valvular defect of the heart — 2 patients had aortic regurgitation; 1 with aortic stenosis experienced dizziness when doing violent aerobatics; 1 had mitral stenosis. The remaining 6 had disorders of rhythm, 3 paroxysmal tachycardia, 1 paroxysmal atrial flutter accompanied by varying heart block, 1 atypical bundle branch block, and 1 'numerous extrasystoles'.

Rook [1947] considered fatigue to have been the principle cause of attacks of unconsciousness in 18 cases. A warrant officer had a number of fainting spells, all associated with an urticarial rash, sometimes also with swelling of the face. The rash could be produced by violent exercise. In some instances attacks of fainting had been so provoked.

Impaired consciousness in 208 pilots and air crews was recorded as primarily emotional in origin. Of these 15 were diagnosed as 'due to panic states', 117 to 'emotion', 49 to 'emotion after stress', 16 to hyperventilation. 'One pilot, whenever he was faced with a difficulty in the air, got into a state in which his mind was a complete blank and for a period he could neither move nor think. How he managed to do 40 h flying without killing himself is difficult to understand'.[7]

7   See appendix 6.

Spontaneous subarachnoid hemorrhage during flight. In 1945 Rash and Goldys published a paper entitled 'Spontaneous Subarachnoid Hemorrhage in a Pilot during Flight'. A 22-year-old fighter pilot instructor was completing a 1-h routine test flight in a P-40 plane when an unheralded attack of unconsciousness occurred, following a sudden, sharp, severe pain in the occipital region during a tight let-down spiral preparatory to landing. According to eye witnesses he landed badly and almost collided with another aircraft, got out of the plane unassisted but was noted to be ataxic and stumbling into objects and people. He was brought to the Base Dispensary and later on recalled that he had at that time severe headache and been nauseous. While being transported from the Dispensary to the Station Hospital in an ambulance, he was unable to move the left side of his body.

Physical examination at the hospital revealed dysarthric speech, a mild lateral nystagmus to the right, and deviation to the left of the protruded tongue. The left side of the body was anesthetic to touch and pain; left leg and arm were paretic and spastic. All tendon reflexes were hyperactive. On the right side, a positive Babinski phenomenon as well as ankle clonus could be elicited. A diagnosis was made of spontaneous subarachnoid hemorrhage presumably from a ruptured intracranial aneurysm. A lumbar tap yielded grossly bloody cerebro-spinal fluid.

During the ensuing week the condition improved and the patient regained alertness and orientation. However, after 3 months, there was still in evidence a left homonymous hemianopia with sparing of the macula, spastic and unsteady gait, and atrophy of the muscles of the left extremities; reflexes were hyperactive, and positive Babinski, Chaddock Gordon and Oppenheim signs could be elicited.

The question was considered whether negative radial acceleration forces during flight (estimated to have amounted to $+ 4\,g$ at the time of the accident) causing a critical rise of intracranial pressure could have initiated the cerebral hemorrhage.[8]

Idiopathic spontanous pneumothorax. A rare kind of unheralded sudden incapacitation of flying personnel results from sudden idiopathic spontanous pneumothorax. Its occasional occurrence in athletes was described in 1947 by Jokl ('Syncope in Athletes', Monograph, 1947). In 1967 Fuchs of the USAF School of Aerospace Medicine, Brooks Air Force Base,

---

8   For a discussion of the cardiovascular problem, see E. Jokl, Textbook of aviation medicine (Unie Volkspers, Capetown 1942); and Medical aspects of aviation, acceleration and deceleration in flight (Pitman, London 1943).

Texas, reviewed the literature on idiopathic spontaneous hemothorax in seemingly healthy military personnel (Publ. 4-67). He referred to one case relating to a 34-year-old B-47 aircraft observer with recurrent episodes of spontaneous pneumothorax in the low pressure chamber at simulated altitudes of between 12,000 and 15,000 ft; to another concerning 29-year-old pilot who suffered and attack while performing a power dive. A third episode occurred in a 27-year-old pilot with 5 years of flying experience who developed idiopathic spontaneous pneumothorax during a fast descent; in a fourth patient, a 34-year-old pilot with 1,780 h of military flying time roentgenological examination in the altitude chamber revealed blebs in the right upper lobe which expanded during simulated ascents.

The onset of idiopathic spontaneous pneumothorax may be sudden, accompanied by pain, dyspnea, cyanosis, and shock causing acute incapacitation of the pilot.

Bleeding peptic ulcer in 19-year-old aviation cadet. SIEGEL and OVERHOLT [1945] described the case history of a 19-year-old USAF cadet who was actively engaged in routine training. His flight instructor reported that the cadet's proficiency in operating his aircraft had suddenly regressed, so much so that 3 consecutive entries had to be made in his record referring to 'improper coordination, bad judgement and increased tenseness'.

It was subsequently established that the young aviator had for some weeks been aware of vague upper abdominal distress, dizziness, spells of perspiration and faintness, and that he had passed black stools. However, because of his desire to graduate with his class, he continued to fly and to practise solo aerobatics, including snap rolls, loops, slow rolls, spins and dives. At no time before or during this period did he experience blackouts, scotomata or dyspnea while flying, even though the anamnesis taken some time later revealed that he had been so weak that he was barely able to get to and from his plane, wearing his flying suit and parachute. It was only after one morning he fainted in his bedroom that he reported sick.

Laboratory studies showed a hemoglobin of 33% (5.2 g) and a red blood count of 2,000,000. Stool examination yielded at 4+ reaction for occult blood. A diagnosis of silent bleeding ulcer was made. When bleeding had ceased under treatment, gastro-intestinal studies demonstrated a deformed, irritable, poorly-filled spastic duodenal bulb.

Appendicitis as presumed cause of crash. The following case was described by SIEGEL and MOHLER [1969]: A fatal Cessna 172 accident in Montana occurred when the pilot apparently got into rising terrain in mountainous conditions and could not climb out of a ravine. The *post-mortem* revealed that the pilot exhibited acute suppurative appendicitis with peri-appendicitis and abscess formation. The Regional Flight Surgeon felt that the attempted gain of altitude and concomitant gas expansion in the appendix and abscess could have caused enough pain to impair the pilot's performance.

Sickling phenomenon and splenic infarction. In 1950 SULLIVAN described the case of an 18-year-old negro soldier who developed nausea, vomiting and left upper abdominal pain while flying. Examination revealed an enlarged tender spleen, sickling of red cells and leucocytosis. During the ensuing years, the same clinical picture was observed during flight by several other investigators. It almost invariably concerned apparently healthy negro personnel. Pronounced left upper quadrant tenderness, paralytic ileus, fever as high as 104° and leucocytosis were the leading symptoms. In most cases enlarged and infarcted spleens (weighing up to 810 g) were removed by surgery. In some instances, old as well as fresh infarcts were discovered. The major splenic arteries were not occluded; but sickling of red cells was always demonstrated in the peripheral blood or in the spleen.

SMITH and COOLEY [1955] undertook an electrophoretic study of blood from 15 persons who had developed splenic infarcts during flight. They found S hemoglobin in every specimen; in 3 cases also C hemoglobin. In the remaining 12, normal A hemoglobin was present inn addition to the S component. Four subjects were anemic. In 3 of them, the anemia was combined with sickle cell trait.

8% of American negroes have sickle cell trait. However, it is sickle cell-hemoglobin disease that renders those afflicted by it prone to splenic infarction in flight. Sickle cell-hemoglobin disease develops on the basis of inheritance of both a gene for sickling and one for hemoglobin. Persons who have only sickle cell trait are less frequently affected though they may also present clinical manifestations, ranging in severity from benign to serious, such as recurrent gross hematuria and fatal diffuse brain disease due to occlusion of small blood vessels by masses of sickled cells. Why organs other than the spleen are not the sites of vascular occlusion due to sickling during flight is not clear. No person with sicle cell hemoglobin S should be allowed to fly. As routine, tests to detect sickling, including electrophoresis of hemoglobin must be employed.[9]

9   The issue is of major relevance to normal and pathological physiology of exercise, a statement which applies to sicke-cell trait alone and more so as collateral finding to atherosclerotic coronary disease. JONES, BINDER and DONOWHO described the autopsy findings of a 21-year-old negro soldier who had died during a physical training session. Marked coronary atherosclerosis was in evidence. There was sickling of all red blood cells. Hemoglobin electrophoresis revealed SA hemoglobin [New Engl. J. Med., *1970:* 323–325].

Epidemiological considerations. Epidemiologically, the problem of sudden cardiac death associated with exercise differs from that of sudden cardiac death unassociated with exercise in that up to the time of the fatal breakdown most victims belonging to the first of the above 2 categories remain free of clinical evidence of cardiac disease and in that their physical performance capacity stays unimpaired.

The same distinction also applies to the broader entity of 'Sudden and Unexpected Death', i.e. death from causes not confined to those associated with diseases of the cardiovascular system: The evidence supporting this statement stems from autopsy studies with different populations, e.g. those conducted by MORITZ and ZAMCHECK [1946] with US soldiers; by BECKER [1952] with subjects in whom pre-existing undiagnosed diseases had caused fatal industrial and automobile accidents; by KULLER et al. [1966] with city dwellers 20 to 39 years old 'who had not been restricted to their homes, to hospitals, or institutions, or unable to function in the community for more than 24 h prior to death'; by LUKE and HELPERN [1968] with subjects between the ages 20 and 45 who had been 'free enough of significant symptomatology not to have sought prior medical attention'; and by JOKL et al. [1966] with athletes who died in association with exercise. Analysis of these data reveals different morbidity patterns. There is a complete absence in the athletes of the 'potentiating direct and indirect effects of acute and chronic alcoholism on natural disease processes of all types', which, according to LUKE and HELPERN [1968], constitute 'major contributing causes of sudden unexpected death' among unselected populations. Likewise, acute infectious diseases rank lower among factors of the initiation of sudden and unexpected fatalities in JOKL's group than in the populations studied by BECKER [1952], KULLER et al. [1966] and LUKE et al. [1968]. The reason is that if an athlete is afflicted by an acute infection, he is likely to be aware of the fact and therefore to abstain from training and competing.[10]

While it is probable that epidemiological studies of sudden and unexpected deaths of pilots will eventually allow identification of pathogenetic patterns of their own, clinical and autopsy data so far available do not render such identification possible. Differential epidemiological subanalyses of this kind could contribute to the understanding of the patho-physiological trigger mechanisms that are involved in the initiation of syncope, with special consideration of the differential diagnosis of causes of episodes of unconsciousness, confusion and amnesia while flying. The 4 primary conditions

---

10   See appendix 7.

found in our *post-mortem* analyses to underlie sudden unexpected cardiac deaths of athletes are: (1) atherosclerotic coronary heart disease with or without myocardial involvement, (2) congenital malformation of coronary arteries or aortic orifice, (3) myocarditis, (4) cardiac tumors.

The requirements for piloting aircraft differ, of course, from those with which ex definitione athletes must comply. We therefore cannot say whether clinical patterns of morbidity and syncope resulting in sudden cardiac deaths of pilots are synonymous.[11]

An analysis of 'Physician Flight Accidents' was reported in 1966 by MOHLER*et al.*, covering the period 1964–1965 during which more than 30 US physicians sustained fatal injuries while piloting light aircraft. The fatality record for the small sample was 4 times the ratio of physician pilots in the general US aviation pilot population. 'Lack of proficiency' represented the primary cause of the crashes in 2, a contributory cause in 5 cases; corresponding incidence rates for 'alcohol' were 1 and 2. In one case there was a history of 'vertigo on previous flights'; in another of drug addiction as well as the following toxicological findings: 3.54 mg% barbiturate (phenobarbital) in the urine, and 2.62 mg% meprobamate in the urine. A syringe was found on the pilot's body and numerous narcotics were recovered from the airplane. The paper by MOHLER *et al.* contains no autopsy data.

Summary

Fatal attack of angina pectoris in military pilot — Myocardial infarction in 34-year-old aviator — Effect of altitude on coronary heart disease — Autopsy studies of coronary arteries of 222 military aviators — Incidence of coronary artery disease in young adults — Cardiovascular system of aging pilots — Relevance of *post-mortem* findings of coronary artery disease in the evaluation of unexplained aircraft accidents — Electrocardiographic studies of flying personnel — Prognostic significance of abnormal T wave in fighter command-pilot — Comparison of rates of incidence of coronary artery disease in RAF and USAF — *Post-mortem* findings in aircraft accident victims who had military flight status — 1965 Bethesda Conference on 'Standards of Physical Fitness of Aircrew' — Heart disease and flying status — Prognostic value of exercise capacity in the assessment of coronary risk after myocardial infarction — Routine medical examination of pilots — 'Aviator's cancer' — 'Relatively sudden deaths' in airline pilots — Cardio-

---

11   See appendix 8.

logical criteria for evaluation of flying status — The role of exercise in the elicitation of sudden fatal collapse — Contributing causative factors — Genetic determinants of onset of fatal collapse in association with strenuous physical exertion — 'Terminal trigger mechanisms' — Episodes of unconsciousness, confusion and amnesia while flying — Impairment of consciousness in RAF personnel during World War II — Spontaneous subarachnoid hemorrhage during flight — Bleeding peptic ulcer in 19-year-old aviation cadet — Sickling phenomenon and splenic infarction — Epidemiological considerations.

References

ANDREWS, P. A. J. and MICHAELS, P.: Nasopharyngeal carcinoma in Canadian bush pilots. Lancet *xiii:* 85–87 (1968).

BECKER, T.: Krankheiten als Mitursachen von tödlichen Verkehrs- und Betriebsunfällen. Mschr. Unfallheilk. *55:* 321–332 (1952).

BENSON, O. O., jr.: Coronary artery disease. Report of fatal cardiac attack in pilot while flying. J. Aviation Med. *8:* 81–84 (1937).

CATHERMAN, R. L.; DAVIDSON, W. H., and TOWNSEND, F. M.: Coronary artery disease in military flying personnel. Aerospace Med. *33:* 1318 (1962).

CATLETT, G. F. and KIDERA, G. J.: Response to carbohydrate loading as a criterion in commercial pilot selection. Aerospace Med. *36:* 554 (1965).

CIVIL AERONAUTICS BOARD: Aircraft Accident Report. (American Flyers Airline Corporation, L-188C, N 183H, Ardmore, Okla., April 22, 1966; Washington, D.C., April, 4, 1967).

CLUVER, E. H. and JOKL, E.: Sudden death of a rugby international after test game. Amer. Heart J. *24:* 405–409 (1942).

COOLEY, J. C.; PETERSON, W. L.; ENGEL, C. E., and JERNIGAN, J. P.: Clinical trial of massive splenic infarction, sicklemia trait, and high altitude flying. J. amer. med. Ass. *154:* 111–113 (1954).

COOPER, K. H.: Heart disease and flying status: Report of a case. Aerospace Med. *38:* 964–967 (1967).

DENNEY, M. K. and READ, R. C.: Scuba-diving deaths in Michigan. J. amer. med. Ass. *192:* 220–222 (1965).

DILLE, J. R. and MOHLER, S. R.: Drug and toxics hazards in general aviation. (Federal Aviation Administration, AM 68–16, Sept. 1968).

ENOS, W. F.; HOLMES, R. H., and BEYER, J.: Coronary disease among US soldiers killed in action in Korea. J. amer. med. Ass. *152:* 1090 (1953).

FINDLAY, G. M.: BOULTER, E. A., and MACGIBBONS, C. B.: A note on sickling and flying. J. roy. Army M. Corps *89:* 138–141 (1947).

GLANTZ, W. M. and STEMBRIDGE, V. A.: Coronary artery atherosclerosis as a factor in aircraft accident fatalities. J. Aviation Med. *30:* 75 (1959).

GRAYBIEL, A. and MCFARLAND, R. A.: Myocardial infarction in a young aviator: Case report illustrating the value of 'routine' electrocardiography in examination of pilots. J. Aviation Med. *12:* 183–193 (1941).

HELLERSTEIN, H. K. and TURELL, D. J.: The mode of death in coronary artery disease, an electrocardiographic and clinicopathological correlation, in sudden cardiac death, pp. 17–37 (Grune and Stratton, New York 1964).

HENDERSON, A. B. and THORNELL, H. E.: Observations on the effect of lowered oxygen tension on sicklemia and sickle cell anemia among military flying personnel. J. lab. clin. Med. *31:* 769–776 (1946).

JAMES, T. N.; FROGGATT, P., and MARSHALL, T. K.: Sudden death in young athletes. Ann. intern. Med. *67:* 1013–1021 (1967).

JOKL, E.: Über einen spontanen Todesfall beim Sport. Schweiz. med. Wschr. *63:* 49–1280 (1933). — Plötzlicher Sporttod durch Myokarditis bei Gonorrhoe. Z. Haut-GeschlKr. *13:* 212–213 (1952). — Sudden non-traumatic death associated with physical exertion, with special reference to drowning. Medicina dello Sport *1:* 11–34 (1964).

JOKL, E. and GREENSTEIN, J.: Fatal coronary sclerosis in a boy of ten years. Lancet *ii:* 659 (1944).

JOKL, E.; MCCLELLAN, J. T., and ROSS, G. D.: Congenital anomaly of left coronary in young athletes. Cardiologia *49:* 253–258 (1966).

JOKL, E.; MCCLELLAN, J. T.; WILLIAMS, W. C.; GOUZE, F. J., and BARTHOLOMEW, R. D.: Congenital anomaly of the left coronary artery in young athletes. J. amer. med. Ass. *182:* 572–573 (1962).

JOKL, E. and MELZER, L.: Acute fatal non-traumatic collapse during work and sport. Sth afr. J. med. Sci. *5:* 4–14 (1940).

KULLER, L.; LILIENFELD, A., and FISHER, R.: Sudden and unexpected death in young adults: an epidemiological study. J. amer. med. Ass. *198:* 248–252 (1966).

LAMB, L. E. (ed.): Symposium on cardiology in aviation. Amer. J. Cardiol. *1:* 1–231 (1960).

LANE, J. C.: Frequency of examination for airline pilots. Aerospace Med. *38:* 736–739 (1967).

LUKE, J. L. and HELPERN, M.: Sudden and unexpected death from natural causes in young adults: Review of 275 consecutive autopsied cases. Arch. Path. *85:* 10–17 (1968).

MANNING, G. W.: An electrocardiographic study of 17,000 fit young Royal Canadian Air Force aircrew applicants. Amer. J. Cardiol. *1:* 70–75 (1960).

MASON, J. K.: Pre-existing disease in aircrew; in Aviation accident pathology: a study of fatalities, p. 179 (Butterworth, London 1962).

MOHLER, S. R.; FREUD, S. F.; VEREGGE, J. E., and UMBERGER, E. L.: Physician flight accidents. Report No. AM 66-25. (Federal Aviation Agency, Office of Aviation Medicine, Aeromedical Applications Division, Washington, D.C., 1966).

MONGE, C. M. and MONGE, C. C.: High altitude disease (Thomas, Springfield, III., 1966).

MORITZ, A. R. and ZAMCHECK, N.: Sudden and unexpected natural deaths of young soldiers: Diseases responsible for such deaths during World War II. Arch. Path. *42:* 459–494 (1946).

O'BRIEN, J. G.: Subarachnoid hemorrhage in identical twins. Brit. med. J. *i:* 607–609 (1942).

ORLADY, H. and CARTER, E. T.: Medical disability in US airline pilots. Unpublished Report. (Airline Pilots Association and Mayo Clinic, 1966).

PUGH, L. G. C.: Deaths from exposure on four inns walking competition 1964. Lancet *i:* 1210–1212 (1964). — Accidental hypothermia in walkers, climbers, and campers. Brit. med. J. *i:* 123–129 (1966).

RASH, J. O. W. and GOLDYS, F. M.: Spontaneous subarachnoid hemorrhage occurring in a pilot during flight. J. Aviation Md. *16:* 91–95 (1945).

REIGHARD, H. L. and MOHLER, S. R.: Some aspects of sudden incapacitation in airmen due to cardiovascular disease. Aerospace Med. *1967:* 1273–1276.

RIGAL, R. D.; LOVELL, F. W., and TOWNSEND, F. M.: Pathologic findings in the cardio-vascular systems of military flying personnel. Amer. J. Cardiol. *1:* 19–25 (1960).

ROOK, A. F.: Fainting and flying. Quart. J. Med. *63:* 181–209 (1947).

SCHREUDER, O. B. and CONSTANTINO, J. G.: Cardiovascular system of the aging pilot. Amer. J. Cardiol. *1:* 26–29 (1960).

SEIPEL, J. H. and WENTZ, A. E.: Unsuspected neurological disease in aviation personnel. A survival following seizures in flight. I and II Aerospace Med. *34* (1963).

SIEGEL, P. V. and MOHLER, S. R.: Medical factors in US general aviation accidents (Federal Aviation Administration, AM-69/2, 1969).

SIEGEL, M. B. and OVERHOLT, B. M.: Bleeding peptic ulcer in a young aviation cadet. Ann. int. Med. *22:* 287–290 (1945).

SMITH, E. W. and CONLEY, C. L.: Sicklemia and infarction of the spleen during aerial flight; electrophoresis of the hemoglobin in 15 cases. Johns Hopk. Hosp. Bull. *96:* 35–41 (1955).

SULLIVAN, B. H., jr.: Danger of airplane flight to persons with sicklemia. Ann. intern. Med. *32:* 338–342 (1950).

SURAWICZ, B. and PELLEGRINO, E. D. (ed.): Sudden cardiac death. Proceedings of Univ. of Kentucky Symposium, Lexington, Ky., October 4–5, 1963 (Grune and Stratton, New York 1964).

WEBSTER, J. G. and HOFFMAN, A. A.: Current concepts of coronary artery disease in a young aircraft population. Conference Report -- Standards of Physical Fitness of Aircrew. Amer. J. Cardiol. *18:* 637–640 (1966).

WILLIAMS, D. J.: Episodes of unconsciousness, confusion, and amnesia while flying; in Psychological disorders in flying personnel of the Royal Air Force investigated during the War 1939–1945. Air Publication 3139. (His Majestys' Stationery Office, London 1947).

WILLIAMS, L. N.: Diabetic airline pilot. Letter to the Editor. Lancet, July 9, 1966.

Authors' address: University of Kentucky, *Lexington, KY 40506* (USA)

Appendices

1. An editorial article in the Amer. J. Cardiol. [November 1968, p. 749] stressed that men of over 60 years of age with heart disease or peripheral vascular disease invariably have several other significant illnesses, usually some degree of emphysema, chronic bronchitis (almost a certainty if they have smoked for many years), generalized arteriosclerosis,

or hypertension. They may have an enlarged prostate gland, glaucoma, cerebrovascular insufficiency, mental disturbances, cholelithiasis, hiatal hernia, diverticulosis or diverticulitis, visual disturbances, insomnia, poor dental health, diabetes, or other impairments in endocrine function.

2. A paper by SIEGEL and BOOZE, Jr., 'A retrospective analysis of aeromedical certification denial actions, January 1961–December 1967' [Federal Aviation Administration, Office of Aviation Medicine, Washington, D.C., May 1968, Report No. Am 68–9] contains a table with numbers of subjects classified into pathological categories, justifying denial of medical certification of 5,727 US airmen during the period January 1961 and December 1967. The most common diagnostic entities were (a) cardiovascular, (b) 'miscellaneous' (including alcohol and drugs, endocrinopathies, general systemic conditions, and administrative denials for failure to provide sufficient medical information on conditions mentioned in the application), (c) nervous and mental, (d) eye and deficient vision, and (e) abdominal.

Less than 1% of all applications (0.79%) were denied. The rate among female applicants was virtually the same as among males. The average age of denied airmen (37.5 years) exceeded the average age of active airman population (35.0 years).

Pathological series	Total	Percent of total
Eye	263	7.86
Ear, nose, throat	80	2.39
Respiratory system	62	1.85
Cardiovascular system	1,289	38.50
Abdominal	195	5.83
Nervous and mental	661	19.74
Bones and joints	48	1.43
Muscles	18	0.54
Miscellaneous Defects	732	21.86
Total	3,348	100.00

3. A recent review of the patho-physiological mechanism underlying sudden cardiac standstill has been given by M. KOERNER in a monograph entitled 'Der plötzliche Herzstillstand' [Springer, 1967].

4. In a publication, 'The safety performance of UK airline operators' [H. M. Stationery Office, London 1968], a number of physiological and clinical aspects of the problem were discussed, among them crew fatigue, which was mentioned as a factor in 4 official reports on accidents, all of them involving independent operators. However, it was not possible to assess the number of occasions on which fatigue might have been a factor in other accidents since the necessary information was not available.

The editor of 'The Lancet' in commenting on the above publication pointed out [June 22, 1968, p. 1358] that no details were given of the 4 accidents under reference even though 4 major crashes could cost the lives of 400 people or more. In at least 1 of the accidents, he writes, there was considerable concern about the length of time the captain had been without sleep. How many of the accidents classified under the headings 'poor judgment or lack of pilot discipline', 'pilot competence', 'lack of crew coordination', or even 'aerodrome deficiency', he asks, had their roots simply in tiredness? 'Surely the possibility is worth at least a recommendation that the necessary information will be forthcoming in future? We may eventually be able to judge whether the pilot of a passenger aircraft is not as liable to fatigue as a long-distance lorry-driver: the President of the Board of Trade may find that a tour of duty, which the Ministry of Transport believes unsafe for the roads, may also be unsafe for the air.'

5. After a solo flight, a pilot under tuition brought his machine to land successfully. Since he failed to taxi over to the tarmac, the mechanics ran out to see if he was in trouble and found him unconscious in the cockpit. The question of epilepsy was raised, but was indignantly repudiated by the pilot, who ascribed the attack to carbon monoxide poisoning. Exhaustive tests failed to show the presence of any appreciable amount of this gas in the machine. The matter remained a mystery until a few days later a typical epileptic fit was observed while the pilot was under observation in a hospital.

ZIVIN and MARSAN studied the 'Incidence and prognostic significance of "epilepti-form" activity in the EEG of non-epileptic subjects' [Brain 91: 751–778 (1968)]. Out of 6497 unselected non-epileptic patients receiving EEG examinations at the National Institute of Neurological Diseases and Blindness, Bethesda, Md. 142 (2.2%) were found to have 'epileptiform' discharges (EDs). Follow-up observations revealed in this group a significantly high incidence of congenital and perinatally acquired brain damage, brain neoplasms, cranial operations, mental retardation, biochemical disorders and treatment with anti-neoplastic agents and steroids. Twenty patients (14.1%) developed seizures.

A history of fainting attacks is of special importance for the evaluation of the medical status of pilots. GOWER's statement, that 'all symptoms or combinations of symptoms that occur in a grand mal attack can also result from cerebral anemia', must be recon-sidered in the light of the hypoxic collapses that occurred during the 1968 Mexico City Olympic Games [JOKL, New Engl. J. Med. June 19, 1969: 1420]. A precise differential diagnosis between cerebrally and cardially elicited seizures accompanied by loss of consciousness has become possible through studies of athletes with congenital heart block [TORKELSON and JOKL, J. Ass. phys. ment. Rehabilitation, March-April, 1967: p. 54–55]. In its asymptomatic form the syndrome differs categorically from that of the A-V block which causes Adams-Stokes seizures. Seizures are conspicuous by their absence in the athletes under reference. M. LEV, who introduced a method for the histopathological study of atrioventricular nod bundle and branches [Arch. Path. 52: 73–83 (1951)], has pointed out that a distinction has to be made also between A-V block of truly congenital origin, and acquired lesions of node, and bundle. Such lesions, he emphasized, can be established already in utero [Amer. J. Cardiol. February, 1967: 266–274]. That among congenital lesions causing A-V block important differences have to be made as regards their clinical relevance has been shown by GREEN et al., (p. 166) whose findings corroborate the validity of the statement that a history of fainting attacks must always be considered to be of cardiological relevance.

6. The Office of Aviation Medicine of the US Federal Aviation Administration published in April 1968 a paper by HIGGINS et al. on 'Effects of two antihistamine-contain-ing compounds upon performance at three altitudes' [E. A. HIGGINS, A. W. DAVIS, Jr., V. FIORICA, P. F. IAMPIETRO, J. A. VAUGHAN, and G. E. FUNKHOUSER, April 1968, 9 pp.

Report No. AM 68-15]. The paper describes a study with 45 human subjects, which showed that the antihistamine phenindamine did not statistically impair performance on a modified Mashburn coordinator, an experimental device used to measure sensory perception and neuro-muscular skill. Another compound which contained the anti-histamine chlorpheniramine did impair performance. Performance was also impaired by increasing altitudes. The combined effects of the chlorpheniramine and exposure to altitude proved more detrimental than the sum of the decrements that each of the above-mentioned influences caused separately. Undesirable side-effects of the phenindamine coupound were also noted.

7. An editorial article in the J. amer. med. Ass. [August 26, 1968, p. 93] on 'Nasal obstruction, a cause of sudden unexpected death?' deals with sudden fatalities in young infants previously well or ill with a minor respiratory infection. Sudden unexpected death accounts for 15,000 fatalities of infants in the United States, twice the number caused by congenital abnormalities. SHAW [Sudden unexpected death in infancy. Amer. J. Dis. Child *116*: 115–119 (1968)] remarked that this loss of young lives with no apparent cause has provoked numerous hypotheses which, however, 'are in large part speculative and unproven'. 'It may very well be', the editor of the J. amer. med. Ass. writes, 'that sudden unexpected death of infants results from different causes or combination of causes that include infections, allergic, anatomic, neurogenic, immunologic, or biochemical components.'

A special issue of the Amer. J. Cardiol. (October, 1968) is devoted to a 'Symposium on sudden death of babies' (Guest Editor Thomas N. James).

8. The medical issue under discussion has received a good deal of attention in reference to automobile traffic hazards. The following is a comment by H. HARTMANN [Triangel, Basel *VII*, 8: 302-307 (1966)] on the problem of syncope occurring without warning at the controls of automobiles.

'This may be no more than a passing faintness, but it may equally take the form of an irreversible circulatory collapse leading to death. The principal heart disorders that can bring about sudden weakness are coronary insufficiency; cardiataxia (especially an inter-mittent block or auricular flutter, where a collapse may be precipitated by an embolism); aortic stenosis; hypotonia (which may be induced by drugs, particularly the ganglionic blocking preparations); myocarditis; aneurysms; and carotid sinus syndrome. Next in importance we should list violent attacks of angina pectoris, which may completely immobilize the patient and thus have serious consequences when the person concerned is driving at the time.'

HARTMANN continues to point out that a very large number of cardiac patients drive a car, quite unaware of their condition. Fatal cardiac crises at the steering wheel do not as a rule occur with dramatic suddenness, and only seldom do they result in substantial injuries to other persons. They are thus in contrast to road accidents due to alcohol, which often have disastrous consequences to others. It is remarkable that a higher than average number of circulatory collapses occur immediately prior to getting into the car, or immediately after finishing a journey. Evidently, the victim often feels the faintness coming on and is able to take suitable action in time. In the case of pilots this is of course difficult or impossible.

The book 'Medical aspects of fitness to drive motor vehicles' [edited by L. G. NORMAN for the Medical Commission on Accident Prevention, Royal College of Surgeons, Lincoln's Inn Fields, London W.C.2], published in 1968, refers to a decision by the

Minister of Transport in Great Britain to grant driving licenses to epileptics who have been free of attacks for over 3 years.

Epilepsy, the editor of 'The Lancet' [June 22, 1968, p. 1359] writes in reviewing the book, is not the only illness which may impair fitness for driving. Heart attacks also pose a risk to other road users. Patients should be told not to drive for 3 months after recovery from infarction, or if their angina is readily provoked while at the wheel. The patient receiving hypotensive therapy should not, he says, drive until his blood pressure is stabilized. Heart block is an unqualified contraindication. Another comment relates to the fact that insulin according to British law is a drug. Thus, a hypoglycemic driver could be found guilty of driving under its influence. Diseases of the eyes and of the central nervous system, and the effects of therapeutic drugs are discussed in detail. A chapter on aging deals with the desirability of routine medical examination for drivers over 60. Too many elderly people, the editor holds, mistakenly insist on continuing to drive. 'Though driving reflexes of a kind seem to survive a long time, the crisis of conscience which these patients cause the family doctor would be eased by regular health checks.'

'Difficulties and dangers caused by boredom, fatigue, and the locomotor disorders are discussed, but not the role of mental disorder. Admittedly, not much is known about this, but some notes on paranoid psychosis would have been helpful. Suicide is probably more often a cause of road deaths than the figures show, and the semi-suicidal behavior of the disordered personality has been described by WILLETT. It is good that the Courts increasingly refuse licenses to accident repeaters.'

9. SIEGEL [US Medicine, January 15 1969] stated that in the United States at the time of compiling his records there were 9884 active pilots over the age of 60 and 869 over the age of 70. A total of 2,640 had no 'useful vision on one eye'. 25,300 pilots are women (see reference to the pharmacological effect of the pill, p. 59).

10. Two important observations belonging to the field of clinical psychology were mentioned by SIEGEL and MOHLER. The first related to a fatal crash, the second to a statistical trend whose analysis may allow further selective prognostications.

A very experienced pilot made a series of low-level flight maneuvers over a river in Hawaii, including a flight under a bridge followed by an abrupt pull-up, in July of 1967. Afterwards he flew to a section of the beach and waved at a girl in a bikini who waved back. The pilot landed on the beach nearby, introduced himself to the girl, then borrowed her telephone, calling several bars to locate his girl friend. While doing so he drank a beer. The pilot then departed saying that if his newly met acquaintance keeps wearing her bikini, he was coming back. He also said, 'Always think happy thoughts'. On becoming airborne he executed two loops near ground level, and on the second loop impacted the ground with fatal consequences. It developed that the pilot had recently separated from his wife and in past years had been known at times as a very heavy drinker. The pilot had also told persons for some time that he was going to fly under the bridge even if it were the last thing he ever did.

The second observation emphasised the importance of accident proneness. During the period 1965–1966, a survey of 15,977 general aviation accidents revealed that 79 pilots experienced 2 or more accidents. 660 had 2 accidents, 62 had 3, and 7 had 4. Within the 'repeater population', 12% were fatal.

11. On behalf of the US Office of Aviation Medicine, J. DILLE and S.R. MOHLER [Report AM 68-16 (1969)] reviewed the evidence concerning 'drugs and toxic hazards in aviation'. Many potent drugs, they point out, can be purchased over the counter; others

are prescribed by physicians who do not inquire about the demands of various occupations; and still others are passed around by well-meaning relatives, friends and neighbors.

It is assumed that drugs have frequently been taken by victims of general aviation accidents but their presence is rarely detected and, even if it is, rarely warrants assignment of a causal role based upon present knowledge. A previous report cited 2 cases where pilots with 3,000 and 8,000 h had human factors accidents and liver barbiturate levels of 0.7 mg % and 0.4 mg %. One of the compounds taken also contained D-amphetamine. Despite known possible effects on judgment of both drugs, no causal role was felt assignable.

The problem lies in predicting the occurrence of undesirable effects. One approach, the military one, is to ban the use of all drugs by aircrew members. This is neither practical nor enforcable in civil aviation. Supervised test doses are useful to determine individual responses. The fact that the condition for which the drug is taken may, in itself, contraindicate flying should be remembered. The fact that performance with drug-relieved symptoms may exceed performance with unrelieved symptons must also be considered.

Some of the medications of greatest use and concern, and some recent accidents involving drugs, as communicated by DILLE and MOHLER are quoted in the original text:

Analgesics. Probably no over-the-counter drug is used more often or more indiscriminately than acetylsalicylic acid. Toxic effects are relatively rare and are almost always associated with large doses. However, gastrointestinal hemorrhage, acute renal failure, blood dyscrasias and idiosyncratic reactions (such as urticaria and angioneurotic edema) are possible. Hemorrhage, when it occurs, is usually due to a competitive antagonism with vitamin K and a decreased circulating prothrombin. A reduced tolerance to hypoxia has been found with salicylates, mostly because of an increase in the metabolic rate.

Analgesic compounds containing aniline derivatives may cause methemoglobinemia if used indiscriminately. Excessive use of bromide-containing compounds may cause psychosis or dermatitis. Quinine-containing preparations may cause vertigo, tinnitus, deafness or nausea.

Of greatest concern is the frequent combination of analgesics, antihistamines and decongestants in compounds which may be taken for analgesic purposes only. The roles of these added ingredients are discussed below.

Antihistamines. Undesirable effects which are possible with the use of antihistamines are drowsiness, inattention, confusion, mental depression, dizziness, decreased vestibular function and impaired depth perception.

Because of the adverse effects of these symptoms on the safety of flight, airmen generally should not take 'short-acting' antihistamines during the 8 h before flight or take the 'long-acting' preparations within 16 h of flying.

Individual consideration should be given to allergic patients who have taken the same drug and dosage for long intervals with a good symptomatic response and no noted side effects.

'Nonsedating' antihistamines (for example, phenindamine tartrate) should be evaluated for their suitability for safe use.

A 38-year-old pilot was killed in a crash of his helicopter due to the improper operation of powerplant and flight controls. He had 2 blood alcohol level determinations reported as 80 and 100 mg % and a 'significant' level of an antihistamine believed to be diphenhydramine. The combined effects of these 2 agents are believed to have caused impaired efficiency and judgment and are given as the cause of the accident.

Antihistamines have also been implicated in a recently reported British accident.

Nasal Decongestants. Since these compounds can occasionally be used to advantage topically during flight (usually for the relief of a blocked eustachian tube during descent), their proper use in flight is not contraindicated. Indiscriminate use of these compounds, particularly by the systemic route, can cause tachycardia, nervousness, tremor, incoordination and mydriasis with visual disturbances.

Motion Sickness Medications. Several types of drugs are used for the relief of motion sickness. Scopolamine, a parasympathetic depressant sometimes used for this purpose, is effective but has sufficient side effects to limit its use. Antihistamines are used widely but often cause drowsiness and dizziness. The sedative antihistamines, such as promethazine, are particularly likely to produce drowsiness. Cyclizine and meclizine also can produce drowsiness and blurred vision may occur with cyclizine. However, side effects are less common with these 2 drugs. Barbiturates have been used but are seemingly of less value and are definitely contraindicated during flight.

Most pilot trainees who become airsick will have no difficulty by the 10th flight. Therefore, cyclizine or meclizine may be temporarily given for motion sickness before training is discontinued, but only under medical supervision, after a test dose, on dual flights and with the consent of the flight instructor. Otherwise, the use of these preparations during flight or within 8 h to 24 h (with meclizine) before flight is generally contraindicated.

Amphetamines. Amphetamines diminish a sense of fatigue, can delay its onset up to 4 h, and 'tend to force the body beyond its natural capacities'. Nervousness, impaired judgment and euphoria are sometimes reported, particularly with overdosage or unusual susceptibility.

Many patients find the stimulation produced by amphetamines pleasant and complain when the physician suggests discontinuance. They can be habit forming and excessive use is common.

When amphetamines are taken in conjunction with a weight reduction program, hypoglycemia may be present. The effects of hypoglycemia are additive to those of hypoxia.

Amphetamines should not be used during flight except in unusual situations (mostly military) in which mission completion is paramount and fatigue represents a greater hazard than drug use during a critical, relatively brief, phase of the flight.

A 35-year-old pilot with 63 h flying time was killed when he crashed while buzzing a tavern at night. He had a blood alcohol level of 200 mg % and a blood amphetamine level of 9 mg %. A 27-year-old pilot with 19.8 h flying time was killed in an unexplained accident. He had a kidney and liver amphetamine level of 0.1 mg % and tissue amobarbital levels of 0.20 to 1.00 mg %. Causal roles were not ascribed to amphetamine in either accident but the frequent presence of more than one drug is demonstrated.

The monoamine-oxidase inhibitors, which are also psychic stimulants, are rarely indicated for persons who are well enough to fly. Significant side effects, particularly hypotension, blurred vision and excitement, also make flying contraindicated. The possible altered response to other drugs and alcohol should be recognized for this group.

Tranquilizers and Sedatives. In most cases, flying is contraindicated by a condition which requires tranquilizers. However, experience has shown that they are prescribed quite liberally and without due concern for the patient's occupation or the undesirable effects of these drugs. While it may not be readily apparent, even the nonsedating tranquilizers usually have some measurable effects on alertness, judgment, efficiency and over-all performance.

Sedatives have been used under controlled conditions by the military to guarantee adequate rest before flight and alertness during flight. Secobarbital sodium, often used for this purpose because it is considered a short-acting sedative, has been found to have effects for up to 8 or 9 h when given in 200-mg doses under controlled experimental conditions.

Pilot duties are contraindicated for 12 to 24 h after the use of sedative agents.

A 50-year-old pilot with 108 h of flying time had a fatal accident when he departed with one passenger on a VFR flight under IFR conditions. He had blood levels of 0.7 mg % of long-acting barbiturate and 40 mg % of alcohol.

A 51-year-old pilot, with 1136 h, and 4 passengers were killed when their aircraft went into a spin at low altitude and crashed. A blood barbiturate level of '0.2 to 0.4 mg %', blood alcohol level of 8 mg %, COHb of 12% and fatigue after a 4-h flight are felt possibly to have been additive and causal.

A 24-year-old pilot with 2203 h was involved in a fatal helicopter crash of undetermined cause. He had a blood phenobarbital level of 0.2 mg % which was not felt to be clinically significant. The reason for drug use was not determined.

A 49-year-old physician was known to use narcotics, barbiturates, and tranquilizers. He had lost his medical license. Erratic behavior had been noted for over 2 years. He had passed out while driving and had had several automobile accidents. A relative, who stopped flying with him, had considered reporting him to the FAA. He had a fatal accident after a stall and spin. He had blood levels of 3.54 mg % of phenobarbital and 0.95 mg % of meprobamate, a combined effect near the stupor level.

A 49-year-old pilot with 100 h of flying time was killed when his plane dived into a reservoir. He had been hospitalized for depression due to alcoholism 2 years before. He had blood levels of 100 mg % of alcohol and 11 mg % of bromide.

Attention is drawn here to the involvement of multiple drug, alcohol and physiologic factors, and the family (and sometimes local official) apathy that is observed too frequently.

Cardiac Agents. Hypertension and most hypotensive agents are disqualifying for flying duties. Medication is the simplest treatment for a physician to render. Where indicated, weight reduction is the treatment of choice. A patient with benign essential hypertension without demonstrable eye, kidney or electrocardiographic changes may not require medication if salt intake is restricted and a controlled weight reduction program is instituted, preferably with exercise. Thereafter, the patient can probably fly safely.

Intermittent drug therapy is not indicated because of the long duration of effects, particularly with reserpine.

Because of the common knowledge that drug relief from disqualifying hypertension is available, a military medical evaluation center analyzes the urine of referred airmen for these agents. Because of the likelihood of a reduction in g-tolerance with these drugs, particularly with the ganglionic blocking agents, their use is of greater concern in military airmen.

In civil aviation, medical certification may be granted for pilots who have taken a hypotensive agent (particularly thiazide diuretics) for a prolonged period and who have demonstrated good control of a relatively stable condition with no significant side effects. Such actions must, of necessity, be on an individualized basis.

A 45-year-old pilot with 91 h entered an unexplained bank and dive just after take-off and he and his passenger were killed. A 0.05 mg % liver level of 'quinine or quinidine' raises the question of a possible medical condition under treatment and inflight incapacitation.

Pilots have had pargyline and other drugs prescribed simultaneously; one such pilot has had an accident due to alcohol. Flying is contraindicated with pargyline and most of the agents which augment its effects and pilots should be advised of this by their physicians; *all patients* should be warned of the possible combined effects.

Muscle Relaxants. These agents, with or without analgesic and tranquilizer actions, cause sufficient weakness, sedation and vertigo to contraindicate pilot duties within at least 12 h after their use.

Steroids. These compounds are often used systemically for the relief of arthritic, allergic, dermatologic and inflammatory conditions which may not, in themselves, contraindicate the performance of pilot duties. Flying is considered contraindicated for 3 days after the systemic use of steroids because of the possible mental changes and other undesirable effects. The topical use of these preparations is not expected to compromise flying safety.

Drugs for Hyperuricemia. These agents are frequently discussed but there is no unanimity of opinion regarding their acceptability for use by flying personnel. The authors are not opposed to the supervised use of uricosuric agents by asymptomatic pilots with hyperuricemia. Headache and gastrointestinal effects, while undesirable, are not usually incapacitating. An attempt should be made to determine the presence and severity of these or other symptoms when these patients are examined for medical certification.

The xanthine oxidase inhibitors are also reported to be effective and relatively free from side effects.

In metabolic diseases like hyperuricemia and diabetes mellitus, where the treatment and not the disease may be disqualifying for flying, pilots and cooperative physicians will often shun treatment. The relative hazards, both immediate and long term, of the treatment vs. the untreated condition must be considered. Long discussions have resulted from such considerations but these are equally inconclusive.

Anticholinergics. Anticholinergic compounds are frequently used and occasionally found associated with aviation accidents and incidents. Since they are frequently combined with sedatives and tranquilizers, their side effects can include, not only blurred vision and ataxia, but sedation, muscle weakness and altered judgment. Their use is contraindicated with flying.

'The Pill'. There are approximately 21,000 active female pilots under the age of 45. We do not know, nor will we probably ever know, the number who take oral contraceptive preparations. Several pilot-physicians who have several patients on these medications have expressed concern over the symptoms of tension noted by many of their patients. While there is insufficient evidence of significant undesirable effects at this time to consider control on their reporting or use by female pilots, we must keep abreast of evolving knowledge on thrombo-embolic, or other, problems with these products and consider these data, age, past medical history, and physical findings in the counseling and certification of these pilots.

Alcohol. There is no generally accepted blood alcohol level, or time after recovery, for the safe operation of an aircraft. The degree to which alcohol increases the effects of hypoxia is similarly inconclusive.

Nystagmic and EEG changes can be noted after the blood alcohol level returns to zero. Decrements in vision and hearing have been reported at levels as low as 10 mg %.

Judgment, comprehension and fine attention are important in flying, and are reduced even at low blood alcohol levels. The incidence of alcohol involvement in fatal accidents is high. Considering individual variation of alcohol effects, the frequent presence of other factors such as drugs and fatigue, no blood alcohol level should be considered compatible with flying.

Pesticides. Aerial application and poisoning through pesticides are a potential cause of accidents. Several cases of poisoning have been admitted to hospitals but remained undiagnosed.

In cases of mild poisoning, rhinorrhea, and salivation are present; constriction of the chest is reported in about 80%; dimness of vision and cough in 60%. Other symptoms are headache, dizziness, twitching, nausea, increased perspiration, fatigue, anorexia, and irritability. In severe poisoning, all these symptoms are increased; also there is vomiting and uncontrollable muscular twitching, in severe cases cyanosis, convulsions, coma, loss of reflexes, and loss of sphincter control. Of diagnostic importance are labels from containers, blood cholinesterase levels, and, in poisoning by parathion and its congeners, urine paranittophenol levels.

Immediate treatment consists of establishing a free air passage, application of artificial respiration, oxygen and when necessary suction. Atropine, given intravenously, is the initial drug of choice. The success of treatment is dependent upon promptness of administration and adequacy of dosage.

Atropine is of little or no value in the treatment of poisoning by the organophosphate compounds. It is contraindicated for pentachlorophenol poisoning, an insecticide which produces symptoms similar to those of the organophosphates, and for chlorinated hydrocarbon poisoning.

Atropine should be administered in dosages of 1 to 2 mg (for mild cases) to 2 to 4 mg (for severe cases), every 5 to 10 min until atropinization occurs (dry flushed skin, pulse rate of 140/min, and pupillary dilatation). 1 g of 2-PAM chloride should be slowly infused, another 500 mg $\frac{1}{2}$ h later if muscular weakness persists.

The patients' clothing should be removed and skin, hair, nails, and eyes decontaminated.

Symptomatic treatment should be continued for 24 to 48 h. A blood sample for cholinesterase determinations should be drawn before 2-PAM is administered. No morphine, tranquilizers, or barbiturates should be given.

Since there are over 55,000 trade name pesticide products in the United States representing over 300 different chemicals it may be appropriate for the physician to call the nearest Poison Control Center for advice.

Chlorinated carbon insecticides vary widely in chemical structure and activity. They affect primarily the central nervous system but may also produce gastrointestinal effects as well as liver and kidney damage. They are stored in fat tissue and released slowly. Convulsions several months after exposure have been observed in animals. Signs and symptoms vary. Headache, nausea, dizziness, hyperexcitability, tremor and in severe cases convulsions are present in most instances. The EEG may show bilateral synchronous spikes, or spike and wave complexes, or slow theta waves.

Carbon Monoxide. Carbon monoxide constitutes up to 2.5% of the volume of cigarette smoke and more in cigar smoke. If the smoke of 3 cigarettes is inhaled in rapid succession a carboxyhemoglobin saturation of 4% may result, reducing visual acuity and dark adaptation to a degree equivalent to the effect of hypoxia produced by an altitude of

8,000 ft. Smoking at 10,000 ft simulates the effects of hypoxia at 14,000 ft. With heavy smoking, carboxyhemoglobin concentrations as high as 8% are possible.

In several aviation fatalities due to fire, carbon dioxide was found to be the immediate cause of death. In 1 case, a 40% carboxyhemoglobin concentration was found. The greatest threat of carbon monoxide poisoning are leakages from defective exhaust systems.

12. An account of 'Studies on Aging in Aviation Personnel', conducted by the Federal Aviation Agency, Washington, D.C., has given in August, 1964, by A. WENTZ (Report No. AM 64-1).

Medicine and Sport, vol. 5: Exercise and Cardiac Death, pp. 64–66
(Karger, Basel 1971)

Fatal Coronary Sclerosis in a Boy of Ten Years

E. Jokl and J. Greenstein

Fatal coronary arteriosclerosis in children is rare. In a study of coronary disease in youths, based on the records of 100 cases in persons under 40 years, Glendy, Levine and White [1937] did not encounter a single example under 20 years and only 8 between 20 and 29 years of age. Master, Dack and Jaffe [1939] analysed 500 case-histories of coronary occlusion; their youngest subject was 27 years old. French and Dock [1944], who reported on 100 fatal cases of coronary arteriosclerosis in soldiers, did not find the disease in subjects under 20, though a large number of younger men are serving with the forces.

A white boy, aged 10 years, collapsed and died 5 min after a boxing match lasting 3 rounds. He had received a number of blows against chest and abdomen but was not knocked down, nor did he seem to be unduly distressed at any time during the fight.

At autopsy the left descending branch of the coronary artery was blocked for a distance of about 1 in, beginning ½ in from the orifice. Above and below the occlusion were slight atheromatous changes in the intima. Histological examination of the diseased portion of the coronary artery revealed an almost complete occlusion. The intima was considerably thickened and hyalinised and a well-organised thrombus occupied almost the whole lumen of the vessel. There was well-marked cellular activity inside the thrombus. Several plaques of calcium were deposited between intima and media and the surrounding tissues were infiltrated with erythrocytes. The internal elastic layer was disrupted and completely absent in parts. No other abnormalities were found in the arterial system. A special effort was made to study the boy's family and previous history, but no light could be thrown on the origin of the condition.

We cannot give an opinion as to the cause of the coronary disease in this case. Nor is it possible to say whether the fist blows which the boy received a few minutes before he died contributed to his fatal collapse.

This latter possibility is suggested by previous observations of injury to the heart in boxing [JOKL, 1941]. NELSON [1941] as well as FRENCH and DOCK [1944] have pointed out that physical activity increases the risk of bleeding into the hypertrophied intima or into atheromatous or calcified plaques in diseased coronary arteries and that such hæmorrhages may expedite fatal collapses in persons thus affected. We therefore feel that the presence of recently extravasated blood in the intima of our young patient's coronary artery is significant. In spite of the fact that the boy's left coronary artery was almost completely occluded, he had been capable of strenuous physical effort immediately before he died.

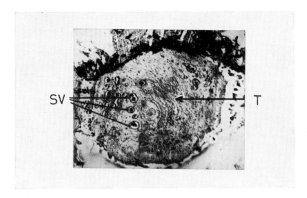

Fig. 1. SV=Small vessels in organizing thrombus; T=Thrombus.

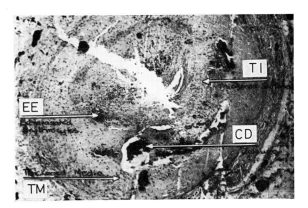

Fig. 2. EE=Extravasated Erythrocytes; TM=Thickened Media; TI=Thickened Intima; CD=Calcium Deposit.

References

FRENCH, A. J. and DOCK, W.: J. amer. med. Ass. *124:* 1233 (1944).
GLENDY, R. E.; LEVINE, S. A. and WHITE, P. D.: Ibid. *199:* 1775 (1937).
JOKL, E.: The medical aspect of boxing (van Schaik, Pretoria 1941).
MASTER, A. M.; DACK, S. and JAFFE, H. L.: Arch. intern. Med. *64:* 767 (1939).
NELSON, M. G.: J. Path. Bact. *53:* 105 (1941).

Authors' address: University of Kentucky, *Lexington, KY 40506* (USA)

Medicine and Sport, vol. 5: Exercise and Cardiac Death, pp. 67–70
(Karger, Basel 1971)

Rheumatic Fever Following Athletic Trauma

E. Jokl and L. Melzer

In 1936 Edstrom reviewed the literature on rheumatic fever following
mechanical trauma. He arrived at the conclusion that injury to a joint can
definitely mobilise a latent rheumatic infarction. The following cases point
in the same direction and raise additional questions.

Case report

Case 1. On the 21st July, 1945, a youth aged 17, while playing football, received a
kick against his right hip. A fortnight later he fell acutely ill and became delirious. There
was neck rigidity and signs of pleurisy and pneumonia, followed by acute endocarditis.
During the ensuing 2 days the patient's temperature rose to 106.6° F and he died. A
history of the deceased was subsequently obtained. The man had been a keen sportsman
and regularly participated in swimming, athletics and games. As a child he had had
whooping cough, measles and chicken-pox and more recently he had suffered from boils
and attacks of sore throat.

Autopsy revealed a hypertrophied left ventricle and a fresh large crumbling thrombotic mass protruding from the ventricular surface of the anterior curtain of the mitral
valve (fig. 1). On examination a small ruptured aneurysm was found beneath the thrombus
that was still attached to the valve. There were also broncho-pneumonic changes in the
bases of both lungs, advanced fatty degeneration of the liver, enlargement and softening
of the spleen, haemorrhage into the paranephric tissue on the right side, multiple infarctions in both kidneys and small haemorrhages in the left frontal lobe of the brain.

This is a case of death due to acute rheumatic fever associated with
infective endocarditis. The disease was apparently mobilised by the football
injury to the right hip. The interval of 2 weeks between the injury and the
manifestations of the fatal disease is typical of cases of this kind. It is

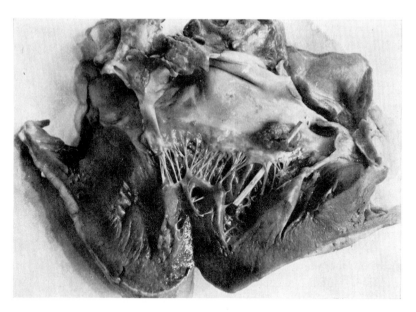

Fig. 1. A large crumbling mass was attached to the ventricular surface of the anterior mitral valve. When the mass was removed, a ruptured aneurysm of the mitral curtain was discovered (match stuck through ruptured aneurysm).

noteworthy that during the final disease the small aneurysm of the mitral valve became the object of a bacterial attack which led to the deposition of a thrombus and subsequently to rupture. A similar mechanism of thrombus formation over a scarred nodule on a mitral valve was seen by SCHMIDT [1939] in a 23-year-old soldier who died after physical exercise. Autopsy revealed fresh blockage by a dislodged part of the thrombus, of the right branch of the coronary artery.

Case 2. A well-known racing cyclist aged 21 fell during a training ride and hurt his left knee. There was no open injury but on the following day the affected joint was swollen. A few days later all the other large joints were swollen and there was a temperature of 104°F. The patient was admitted to hospital where he was told that he suffered from rheumatic fever and that his heart was affected. Within the following 3 weeks the swelling of his joints subsided, his temperature returned to normal, but his heart 'remained bad'. The patient now suffered from 'stitch' in the cardiac region and dyspnoea on slight exertion.

In spite of his disability he tried to continue his bicycle racing but could not do so since he found that his condition had badly deteriorated. Before the accident and the illness that followed it, the patient had been successful in a large number of cycling competitions. On one occasion he covered 160 miles in 7 h, being known in particular for his strength in mountainous territory. A few weeks before his accident he had still participated in a race leading over 140 miles.

His athletic career came literally to a standstill when during a training ride he became sick and had to dismount. He fainted and when he regained consciousness had a headache, felt nauseous and weak, was breathless and had to rest for 1 h before he could go home.

Clinical and X-ray examination revealed a pathologically enlarged heart (fig. 2). The apical beat could be palpated in the 7th intercostal space, 2 in outside the mammilary line and a loud systolic murmur was heard over all ostia. The second pulmonary sound was accentuated. No diastolic murmurs were detected on auscultation. Blood pressure was 100/30. The liver which could be felt 1¼ in below the costal margin was tender on pressure.

Electrocardiographic examination revealed P-Q conduction time of .22 sec. P3 was biphasic, R1 negative. T waves were normal in all leads. The whole picture suggested right preponderance.

It was ascertained that at age 9 the patient had St. Vitus Dance.

This young man then suffered from mitral insufficiency, and his heart muscle was affected. The disease which was of rheumatic origin had developed subsequent to a trauma to the knee. It is important that the patient reports he had suffered from St. Vitus Dance at age 9. He therefore appears

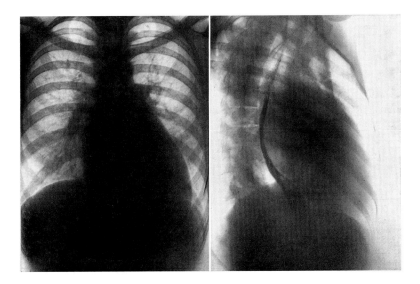

Fig. 2. Mitral insufficiency of rheumatic origin following trauma to joint incapacitating racing cyclist. X-ray examination revealed pathological enlargement of heart, especially to left (antero-posterior view) and bulging of left ventricle posteriorly as indicated by displacement of oesophagus (containing contrast material) in lateral plane.

to have harboured a latent infectious disease which the injury to the knee mobilised. Between ages 9 and 21 he had apparently been healthy and he had excelled in a particularly strenuous sport.

After the severe illness following his fall the patient tried to continue his athletic career. It was the syncope to which reference has been made, rather than the symptons of his cardio-vascular disease, i.e. the dyspnoea, tachycardia, thirst and nycturia that compelled him to seek medical advice. There was no improvement of this man's condition during a period of 5 years subsequent to his coming under medical observation. In contrast to common experiences with hospital patients, many athletes tend to dissimulate existing diseases rather than to exaggerate the importance of, or even simulate illnesses.

Summary

Two cases are presented of trauma to large joints mobilising latent systemic infections leading to acute rheumatic fever with involvement of the heart. In both instances the patients, who had been outstanding athletes prior to being injured, were incapacitated through the illness. The one died and the other remained crippled.

References

EDSTROEM, G.: Mechanisches Trauma und nachfolgende Febris rheumatica. Acta med. scand. 88, 2–4: 342 (1939).
SCHMIDT, W.: Tod durch Coronarembolie aus scheinbar völliger Gesundheit mit Berücksichtigung der Dienstbeschädigungsfrage. Dtsch. Militärarzt, 3: 351 (1939).

Authors' address: University of Kentucky, *Lexington, KY 40506* (USA)

Medicine and Sport, vol. 5: Exercise and Cardiac Death, pp. 71–81
(Karger, Basel 1971)

Traumatic Left Ventricular Aneurysm

Cardiac Thrombosis Following Aneurysmectomy

D. L. GLANCY, PH. YARNELL and W. C. ROBERTS

The usual cause of left ventricular aneurysm is coronary atherosclerosis with transmural myocardial infarction, and one of the rare causes is blunt trauma to the chest. Seven patients with well documented traumatic left ventricular aneurysm have been reported [1–6]; in 5 the aneurysm ruptured between 2 and 90 days after the injury [1–3, 6] and in the other 2 the left ventricular aneurysm persisted [4, 5]. The present report describes a young man with a left ventricular aneurysm that developed following blunt injury to the chest. Multiple systemic emboli occurred, and the aneurysm was resected. Although no thrombus was found in the resected aneurysm, fatal multiple systemic emboli occurred many months postoperatively, and at necropsy a large thrombus was found attached to the left ventricular suture line. The authors know of no previous reports describing left ventricular thrombosis following resection of a cardiac aneurysm under cardiopulmonary bypass.

Report of Patient

The patient was well until November 1962, when at age 20 he was struck in the chest while playing football. Ten minutes later severe substernal and interscapular pain, dyspnea and diaphoresis developed. The pain lasted for 2 days. A month later, intermittent claudication of the left calf and coldness of the left foot developed. In January 1963 numbness, paralysis and pain in both legs suddenly developed, and the popliteal, posterior tibial and dorsalis pedis arterial pulses were found to be absent bilaterally. Warfarin sodium was administered. Several superficial areas of necrosis on the left foot subsequently healed, and the pain at rest and the sensory and motor deficits diminished. An ECG taken in February 1963 showed an anterolateral myocardial infarct of indeterminate age.

When first seen at the Clinical Center in August 1963, the patient was asymptomatic except for claudication of the left leg on walking 5 blocks. The left pedal pulses were absent. The blood pressure was 130/70 mm Hg. Examination of the precordium disclosed no abnormalities. The chest roentgenogram and electrocardiogram are shown in figures 1a and 2a, respectively. The serum cholesterol was normal (190 mg/100 ml), as were the serum phospholipids and triglycerides.

By October 1964 he was able to play touch football without discomfort, and he stopped taking warfarin sodium. Three weeks later he noted transient pain in the right flank, numbness of both legs and coldness of both feet; the arterial pulses in each foot were diminished.

Operative findings and treatment. In June 1965 he underwent cardiac catheterization and cineangio-cardiography at another institution. The pressures were normal, and the left ventriculogram showed an apical aneurysm with paradoxic pulsations and irregular filling defects suggesting the possibility of mural thrombi (fig. 3). Coronary cinearteriography showed normal left circumflex and right coronary arteries but variations in the diameters of the lumens of the distal anterior descending and diagonal branches of the left coronary artery. In July 1965 a cardiac operation under cardiopulmonary bypass was performed. The left ventricular apical wall, measuring approximately 3 by 3 cm, was found to be densely fibrotic and slightly thinned, but only minimal paradoxic motion was observed in it. The central 2 by 2 cm. of this area was excised, and no intra-aneurysmal thrombus was found. The patient's early postoperative course was uneventful, and he was discharged on no medication. $1\frac{1}{2}$ months following the procedure, however, he had a transient episode of numbness of the right side of his tongue and face and clumsiness of the right arm and leg.

Subsequent course. Thereafter, he was well until January 26, 1966, when he was readmitted to the Clinical Center because of the sudden appearance of signs and symptoms diagnostic of brain-stem infarction. A right vertebral arteriogram performed 2 weeks later showed occlusion of the basilar artery. A variety of complications arose during this final illness: inability to handle secretions necessitating tracheostomy; thrombosis at the site of the right brachial arteriotomy requiring thrombectomy; right femoral arterial embolization leading to embolectomy; recurrent cerebral emboli; and gastrointestinal

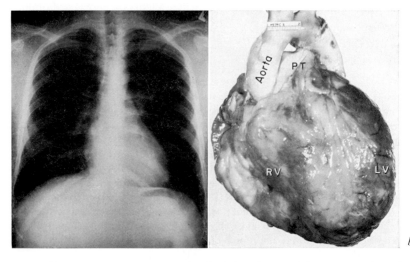

a   *b*

Fig. 1.ᵃ Chest roentgenogram, 15 months after injury, is normal; ᵇ anterior surface of the heart at necropsy. LV = left ventricle; RV = right ventricle; PT = pulmonary trunk.

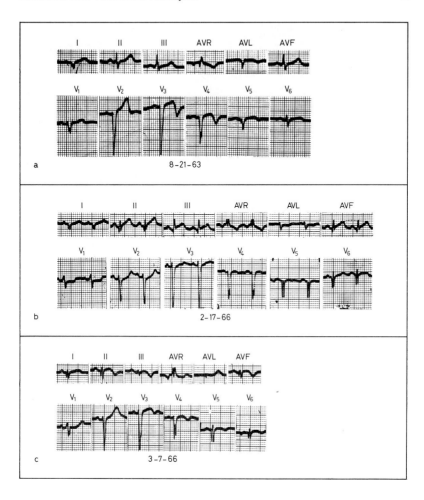

Fig. 2. Electrocardiograms. *a* Aug. 21, 1963, 9 months after injury an anterolateral myocardial infarction of indeterminate age is indicated. ECGs shortly after operation and until 4 months before death were similar; *b* Feb. 17, 1966, 3 months before death, additional changes of acute posteroinferior injury; *c* March 7, 1966, 9 weeks before death, further evolution of the posteroinferior myocardial infarct. At necropsy there was, in addition to the dense anteroapical scar shown in figure 4, extensive, patchy, cellular and acellular fibrosis of the posterior left ventricular wall from apex to base. The generalized circulatory problems experienced by the patient at the time of the acute electrocardiographic changes probably contributed greatly to the posterior wall infarction, since the coronary arteries supplying this area were widely patent.

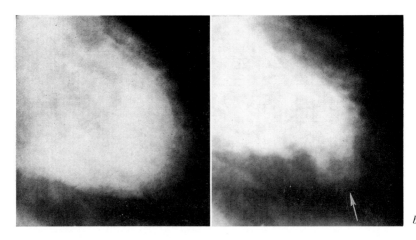

a   *b*

Fig. 3. Left cineventriculograms, right anterior oblique projection. ᵃ Ventricular diastole. The apical aneurysm is not apparent; ᵇ ventricular systole. The arrow points to the apical aneurysm, which bulges paradoxically as the ventricle contracts. The radiolucent filling defect within the aneurysm suggests a possible mural thrombus, but none was found at cardiac operation.

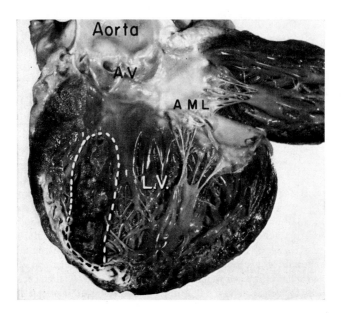

a

Fig. 4. Legend see page 75.

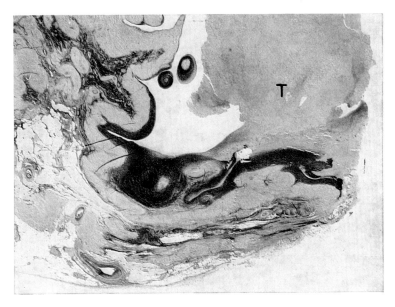

b

Fig. 4. Left ventricular thrombus. *ᵃ* Opened left ventricle. At its apex is a dense fibrous scar, which extends half way up the anterior wall. Attached to the apex is a large mural thrombus enclosed in dashes. AML = Anterior mitral leaflet; AV = aortic valve; LV = left ventricle; *ᵇ* section through the left ventricular apex shows scarring of the free wall and interventricular septum and the attachment of the mural thrombus (T) to the free wall. There is a large amount of elastic tissue, which stains black, in the scar. (Elastic tissue stain, × 5.5 reduced by 31%.)

hemorrhage requiring nine transfusions and cessation of heparin therapy. ECGs during the first 3 weeks of hospitalization were unchanged from those in 1963 (fig. 2b). However, concomitant with the femoral arterial embolization and gastrointestinal bleeding, changes of acute inferior infarction appeared (fig. 2c). On May 11, 1966, the clinical picture of mesenteric arterial occlusion developed, and the next day he died. Numerous tests were done during this admission to determine if this patient had blood constituents which would increase his propensity to form clots, but none were found.

Autopsy. The left ventricular apex of the heart (wt, 330 g) was extensively scarred, and a thrombus was attached to it (fig. 1b and 4c). In addition, there was patchy but extensive scarring of the posterior left ventricular wall. The anterior descending coronary artery was severely narrowed 9 cm from its origin by an organizing and fresh thrombus (fig. 5). The proximal anterior descending and the other major coronary arteries were free of thrombi and atheromata. The midline basilar portion of the pons was necrotic, and the basilar artery was focally occluded by thrombotic material, as were several of the midline perforating branches. There was a fresh thrombus in the superior sagittal sinus and in the superior mesenteric artery 5 cm from its origin. The small intestine was distended and focally infarcted. Infarcts also were found in the kidneys and spleen, and the right femoral artery was occluded by a recent thrombus.

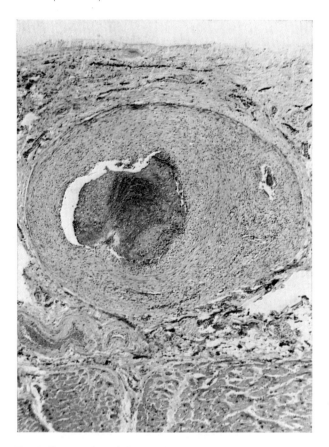

Fig. 5. Cross section of the anterior descending coronary artery 9 cm from its origin. It is almost completely occluded by an organizing and fresh thrombus. Recanalization of the organizing thrombus can be seen in the right half of the photomicrograph. The organized thrombus presumably dates from the time of injury. The fresh thrombus may have arisen *in situ*, perhaps coincident to hypovolemia, or may represent embolic material. (Hematoxylin and eosin stain, × 39 reduced by 8%).

Comments

Nonpenetrating chest trauma is frequently followed by transient clinical, electrocardiographic, or roentgenographic evidence of myocardial or pericardial injury [7, 8] and when fatal, often by cardiac laceration or rupture [2, 8–11] even without overt signs of a chest injury [2, 3, 8, 12]. However, clinically detectable cardiac damage in late survivors of blunt trauma to the chest is unusual, although ventricular septal defect [8], aortic regurgitation [13], ruptured papillary muscle [8], and constrictive pericarditis [14] all have been reported. Myocardial contusion, the most frequent cardiac injury following blunt chest trauma, rarely leaves clinically detectable evidence of cardiac abnormality in those patients surviving the injury by several months [7, 8, 15]. Animal experiments and observations on patients who survived blunt chest trauma, but subsequently died of unrelated diseases, indicate that the myocardial injury heals with little and sometimes no detectable scar [8, 9, 11].

The coronary arteries are relatively resistant to injury by blunt chest trauma. Laceration of these vessels is uncommon, and thrombosis is rare. Of 546 patients with fatal nonpenetrating cardiac trauma reported by Parmley and associates [8], only 10 had lacerations, and none had thrombosis of a coronary artery, despite the frequency of myocardial contusion adjacent to extramural coronary arteries. HAWKES [2] likewise recorded no coronary arterial injuries in 70 autopsy subjects who died of blunt trauma involving the heart. Furthermore, MORITZ [12] found that the coronary arteries of dogs were much more resistant to injury by direct trauma than the adjacent myocardium. Thrombosis of the coronary vessels in these animals was especially difficult to produce, and when it did occur, the vessels were only partially occluded.

Coronary thrombosis due to blunt chest trauma. It is usually exceedingly difficult to establish blunt chest trauma as the cause of coronary arterial thrombosis. Before coronary thrombosis is attributed to trauma alone, ideally 3 criteria should be satisfied: (1) a history of chest trauma which shortly antedates the onset of cardiac signs and symptoms; (2) evidence of damage to the myocardium adjacent to the thrombosed coronary vessel; and (3) absence or near absence of intrinsic disease in the coronary arteries. Utilizing these strict criteria, we have found no reports of patients in whom coronary thrombosis could be unequivocally attributed to blunt chest trauma. In the patient described by JOACHIM and MAYS [4] and in 1 patient (No. 4) described by DEMUTH and ZINSSER [11] chest trauma may have been the sole cause of coronary thrombosis, but insufficient description of the coronary arteries was given to be certain. At least 4 additional patients have been reported in whom blunt chest trauma probably played a contributory role in causing coronary thrombosis [12, 16–18]. Each of these patients, however, had considerable coronary atherosclerosis. Very often patients who receive blunt chest trauma also incur other injuries which cause hypovolemia and shock, and it is possible that these consequences of the injury play a more important role in producing coronary thrombosis than direct injury to these vessels themselves. In the present patient the initial episode of myocardial necrosis, which led to formation of the aneurysm, could have been the direct result of myocardial contusion, the indirect result of traumatic coronary thrombosis, or a combination of these factors.

Mural thrombosis in myocardial contusion and aneurysm. Small mural thrombi frequently develop when the endocardium is contused [8], and systemic embolization occasionally follows. Two of the 546 patients with fatal, nonpenetrating, cardiac trauma described by PARMLEY *et al.* [8] died of thromboembolic complications. HILDEBRANDT's patient [5] suffered blunt chest trauma at age 9 and became hemiplegic shortly before his death at 27; at necropsy a mural thrombus was found within an old left ventricular aneurysm. RANDERATH's [6] 34-year-old patient died 2 days after extensive myocardial contusion, and at necropsy a left ventricular aneurysm containing a mural thrombus and occlusions by emboli of 1 femoral and of 2 coronary arteries were found. PARSONS-SMITH and WILLIAMS [19] described a 15-year-old boy who recovered from myocardial contusion and left hemiparesis, which had developed the day after the contusion.

Postoperative embolization. Systemic emboli are common, however, in patients with chronic left ventricular aneurysms due to coronary atherosclerosis [20] and they constitue one of the indications for operative intervention. Before cardiopulmonary bypass was available, a left ventricular aneurysm was resected by applying a clamp across its mouth and excising the tissue distal to the clamp. As a consequence of this closed procedure, a portion of the mural thrombus frequently was dislodged into the circulation or was not removed, a problem that often led to operative or postoperative systemic embolization [21, 22]. With cardiopulmonary bypass, complete removal of the aneurysm and intra-aneurysmal thrombus became possible. In 51 reported patients who have undergone left ventricular aneurysmectomy under cardiopulmonary bypass, operative and postoperative emboli have not been recorded [23–31].

In retrospect, it would appear that the present patient should have been placed on anticoagulants postoperatively on a long-term basis. Anticoagulation following left ventricular aneurysmectomy is not a common practice of any clinic of which we are aware, but this procedure needs further consideration.

Summary

The clinical and pathologic features of a 23-year-old man with a left ventricular aneurysm that developed following blunt trauma to the chest are described. Systemic emboli occurred both before left ventricular aneurysmectomy under cardiopulmonary bypass was performed and several months following the operation. This complication proved to be fatal. A large mural thrombus in the left ventricle was the apparent source of the emboli.

References

1 FRENCH, H.: A case of traumatic aneurysm of the heart. Guy's Hosp. Rep., *66:* 349 (1912).

2 HAWKES, S. Z.: Traumatic rupture of the heart and intrapericardial structures. Am. J. Surg. *27:* 503 (1935).

3 PITTS, H. H. and PURVIS, G. S.: Ruptured traumatic aneurysm in a child. Canad. med. Ass. J. *57:* 165 (1947).

4 JOACHIM, H. and MAYS, A. T.: Case of cardiac aneurysm probably of traumatic origin. Amer. Heart J. *2:* 682 (1927).

5 WARBURG, E.: Subacute and chronic pericardial and myocardial lesions due to nonpenetrating traumatic injuries, p. 24. Translated by ANDERSEN and SEIDELIN (Oxford Univ. Press, London 1938).

6 RANDERATH, E.: Frühveränderungen des Herzens nach Commotio cordis. Verh. dtsch. Ges. Path. *30:* 163 (1937).

7 BARBER, H.: The effects of trauma, direct and indirect, on the heart. Quart. J. Med. *13:* 137 (1944).

8 PARMLEY, L. F.; MANION, W. C., and MATTINGLY, T. W.: Nonpenetrating traumatic injury of the heart. Circulation *18:* 371 (1958).

9 BRIGHT, E. F. and BECK, C. S.: Nonpenetrating wounds of the heart. Amer. Heart J. *10:* 293 (1935).

10 KISSANE, R. W.: Traumatic heart disease: Nonpenetrating injuries. Circulation *6:* 421 (1952).

11 DEMUTH, W. E. and ZINSSER, H. F.: Myocardial contusion. Arch. intern. Med. *115:* 434 (1965).

12 MORITZ, A. R.: Injuries of the heart and pericardium by physical violence; in Gould Pathology of the heart, 2nd ed., p. 849 (Thomas, Springfield, Ill. 1960).

13 LEVINE, R. J.; ROBERTS, W. C., and MORROW, A. G.; Traumatic aortic regurgitation. Amer. J. Cardiol. *10:* 752 (1962).

14 GOLDSTEIN, S. and YU, P. N.: Constrictive pericarditis after blunt chest trauma. Amer. Heart J. *69:* 544 (1965).

15 ROSE, K. D.; STONE, F., and FUENNING, S. I.: Cardiac contusion resulting from 'spearing' in football. Arch. intern. Med. *118:* 129 (1966).

16 JOKL, E. and GREENSTEIN, J.: Fatal coronary sclerosis in a boy of ten years. Lancet *ii:* 659 (1944).

17 LEVY, H.: Traumatic coronary thrombosis with myocardial infarction. Arch. intern. Med. *84:* 261 (1949).

18 LEHMUS, H. J.; SUNDQUIST, A. B., and GIDDINGS, L. W.: Coronary thrombosis with myocardial infarction secondary to nonpenetrating injury of the chest wall. Amer. Heart J. *47:* 470 (1954).

19 PARSONS-SMITH, G. and WILLIAMS, D.: Cerebral embolism following contusion of the heart. Brit. med. J. *i:* 10 (1949).

20 SCHLICHTER, J.; HELLERSTEIN, H. K., and KATZ, L. N.: Aneurysm of the heart: A correlative study of proved cases. Medicine *33:* 43 (1954).

21 BAILEY, C. P.; BOLTON, H. E.; NICHOLS, H., and GILMAN, R.: Ventriculoplasty for cardiac aneurysm. J. thorac. Surg. *35:* 37 (1958).

22 SULLIVAN, J. J.; MANGIARDI, J. L., and JANELLI, D. E.: Successful resection of ventricular aneurysm. Ann. Surg. *151:* 22 (1960).

23 CHAPMAN, D. W.; AMAD, K., and COOLEY, D. A.: Ventricular aneurysm: 14 cases subjected to cardiac bypass repair using the pump oxygenator. Amer. J. Cardiol. *8:* 633 (1961).

24 EFFLER, D. B.; WESCOTT, R. N.; GROVES, L. K., and SCULLY, N. M.: Surgical treatment of ventricular aneurysm. Arch. Surg. *87:* 249 (1963).

25 LAM, C. R.; GALE, H., and DRAKE, E.: Surgical treatment of left ventricular aneurysms. J. amer. med. Ass. *187:* 1 (1964).

26 LILLIHEI, C. W.; LEVY, M. J.; DeWALL, R. A., and WARDEN, H. E.; Resection of myocardial aneurysms after infarction during temporary cardiopulmonary bypass. Circulation *26:* 206 (1962).

27 CATHCART, R. T.; FRAIMOW, W., and TEMPLETON, J. W.: III. Postinfarction ventricular aneurysm: 4-year follow-up of surgically treated cases. Dis. Chest. *44:* 449 (1963).

28 KAY, J. H.; ANDERSON, R. M.; BERNSTEIN, S., and TOLENTINO, P.: Removal of left ventricular aneurysm with heart exposed and circulation maintained by heart-lung machine. Calif. Med. *92:* 434 (1960).

29 GLENN, W. W. L.; TOOLE, A. L.; LONGO, E.; HUME, M., and GENTSCH, T. O.: Induced fibrillatory arrest in open-heart surgery, New Engl. J. Med. *262:* 852 (1960).

30 NEPTUNE, W. B.; BOUGAS, J. A., and PANICO, F. G.: Open-heart surgery without the need for donor-blood priming in the pump oxygenator. New Engl. J. Med. *263:* 111 (1960).

31 TELLING, M. and WOOLER, G. H.: Excision of cardiac aneurysm. Lancet *ii:* 181 (1961).

Authors' address: Dr. D. L. GLANCY, Dr. P. YARNELL and Dr. W. C. ROBERTS, 478 Peachtree Street N. E., *Atlanta, GA* (USA)

Medicine and Sport, vol. 5: Exercise and Cardiac Death, pp. 81–90
(Karger, Basel 1971)

Death of a Wrestler

E. Jokl and B. Newman

The following is a report of the fatal collapse of an athlete with advanced atherosclerotic coronary artery disease and extensive degenerative myocardial changes.

Case Report

A 45-year-old wrestler complained of pressure in his chest immediately after a match. He died in the dressing room a few minutes later. His wife said that he had competed in wrestling competitions for over 20 years; that he had never been seriously ill; and that he had not complained of symptoms referable to his heart.

Autopsy revealed a heart, weighing 350 g. The left ventricular wall was 1.2–1.3, the right 0.3 cm thick. All valves were normal. The apical region of the posterior wall of the left ventricle contained an area of fibrosis measuring $3 \times 2 \times 1$ cm. The left coronary artery showed severe diffuse atherosclerosis with ulceration. Its ostium was occluded by a semi-firm non-adherent thrombus measuring $0.5 \times 0.4 \times 0.4$ cm. The lumen of the right coronary artery was narrowed by confluent calcified atheromatous plaques.

Microscopic examination (fig. 1) revealed numerous focal areas of myocardial degeneration with patches of complete fibrous replacement. No inflammatory infiltrate was present. The left coronary artery showed advanced widespread intimal atherosclerosis with considerable narrowing of the lumen at different places. Embedded in several atheromatous deposits were cholesterol clefts. There were several areas of calcification. The calcium was precipitated in fine droplet-like concretions. The thrombus showed laminations of fibrin, red cells and leucocytes but no evidence of fibroblastic organization. Advanced localized atherosclerotic changes were seen in the right coronary artery.

In summary, autopsy of a 45-year-old trained athlete who had died after wrestling revealed advanced coronary atherosclerosis and severe myocardial disease. The deceased had been free from symptoms referable

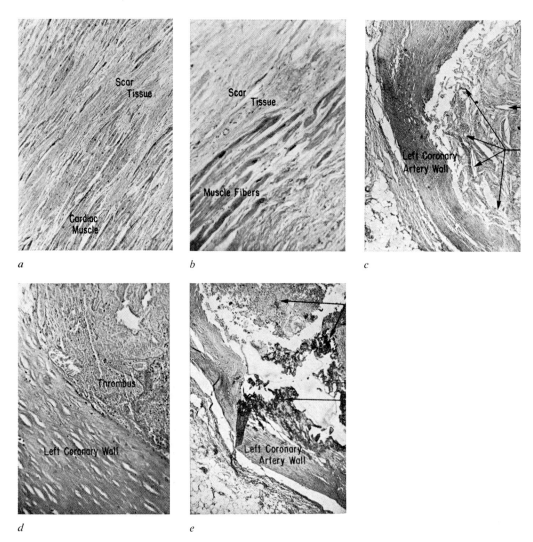

Fig. 1. a: Myocardium with extensive fibrous replacement of muscle, *b:* myocardium with hypoxic degenerative changes in muscle fibers and extensive replacement with fibrous tissue, *c:* left coronary artery wall with atheromatous deposit, *d:* left coronary artery wall and thrombus, *e:* left coronary artery with calcified deposits in atheromatous material.

Hematoxylin and eosin stain. × 100. ST = Scar Tissue, CM = Cardiac Muscle, MF = Muscle Fibers, LCAW = Left Coronary Artery Wall, CF = Cholesterol Cleft, ADL = Atheromatous Deposit in Lumen, T = Thrombus, AD = Atheromatous Deposit, CDI = Calcium Deposit in Intima.

to his heart. His physical performance capacity had been above that of most untrained middle-aged healthy men. In considering the evidence, it seems appropriate to ask whether the strenuous exertion may have been a contributory cause of his sudden death and whether his age could have been a predisposing factor. We shall also comment on several clinical and pathological aspects of fatal collapses in seemingly healthy subjects with coronary and myocardial disease whose exercise tolerance had been unimpaired.

Exercise

BEAN [2], in a study based on 300 autopsies selected from 9,626 consecutive protocols, found that in 44 cases of infarction the onset of symptoms occurred while the patients were at rest, 16 of them being asleep; in 44, during activity, in 14, while the patients were eating; and in 4, while the patients were deeply intoxicated. In a study of 817 attacks or coronary artery thrombosis occurring in 555 patients, MASTER, DACK, and JAFFE [26] found that 21.7% occurred while the patient was at rest, 19.6% while he was asleep, 13.6% during mild activity, 5.3% during moderate activity, and 18% while the patient was walking; thus 41.3% occurred while the patient was at rest or sleeping and 36.9% during mild or moderate activity. In only 2.1% was there a history of unusual or severe exertion. These authors concluded that there is no one factor or group of factors responsible for the onset of an attack of coronary artery thrombosis and that the apparent association of an attack with some external condition is merely coincidental. In another article MASTER, GUBNER, DACK and JAFFE [28] arrived at the same conclusion. In 1941, MASTER, DACK, and JAFFE [27] studied the precipitating factors of the premonitory symptoms of coronary artery occlusions in 70 cases and concluded that effort did not initiate them. However, in 1944, MASTER [29], in defining angina pectoris, acute coronary insufficiency and coronary occlusion, expressed the opinion that acute coronary insufficiency is associated with a precipitating factor which might be either an increased demand for coronary blood flow or anything which actually reduces the flow.

At this stage it had become apparent that the question of the relationship between exercise and sudden death in subjects with advanced ischemic heart disease could be answered only on the basis of epidemiologic studies. An opportunity to conduct such studies offered itself during World War II when the US Army Institute of Pathology collected autopsy reports from military installations throughout the United States and elsewhere. Between

1947 and 1951 MORITZ and ZAMCHEK [33] and YATER *et al*. [42, 43] presented the required evidence derived from combined clinical, pathological and epidemiological analyses of a sufficiently large volume of data.

Among 40,000 autopsy protocols received at the US Army Institute of Pathology between 1942 and 1946, MORITZ and ZAMCHEK found 98 reports of *post-mortem* examinations of young and apparently healthy soldiers who had suddenly and unexpectedly died from coronary atherosclerotic disease. Most of them had passed one or more physical examinations prior to their induction into the Army.

The authors considered that if the onset of acute heart failure due to coronary insufficiency were unrelated to any extrinsic factor, the incidence during any given interval of time throughout the day or the night should be proportional to the duration of that interval. If such were the case and if the soldiers spent an average of $\frac{1}{3}$ of their time sleeping, it might be expected that the onset of acute heart failure would have taken place during sleep in approximately $\frac{1}{3}$ of the deaths. However, the onset of acute heart failure occurred during sleep in only 15% of the cases. In 29% the onset of heart failure coincided with or immediately followed strenuous physical exertion though it was estimated that not more than 17% of the average soldier's 24-h day was devoted to strenuous physical activity. It thus appeared that the number of those whose fatal seizures occurred incident to exertion was in excess of that which would be expected by random distribution. It was in this context that the authors wrote, '*If a young man is to die unexpectedly of coronary disease, the onset of the terminal attack of acute heart failure is more likely to take place during strenuous physical exertion than during sleep.*'

Corresponding results were obtained by YATER *et al.* [42] who reported that the onset of the terminal syncope leading to sudden death of 324 apparently healthy soldiers whose autopsy revealed advanced ischemic heart disease occurred relatively more often during strenuous activity than during mild and moderate activity and sleep. The proportion of attacks occurring during strenuous activity was more than twice as great as the proportion of the time spent in such activity; the proportion during mild and moderate activity was about equal to the proportion of time thus spent; and the proportion of men stricken while asleep was about $\frac{1}{3}$ that of the proportion of time normally spent in sleep.

A disproportionately large number of those who died or who suffered myocardial infarcts were afflicted within one year of entering service. *The rigors of military service also seemed to have been a factor in precipitating the attacks.*

Age

In MORITZ and ZAMCHEK's [33] series no deaths occurred in *soldiers* under 20 years of age though 9% of the total Army personnel belonged to this age category. In the age groups 20–24, 25–29, 30–34, and 35–39, rates of deaths increased out of proportion to their representation in the total Army personnel.

No corresponding age pattern has been encountered in studies on sudden cardiac death of athletes. We have described fatal collapses of 5 youths aged 10, 14, 15, 16, and 17 with silent coronary heart disease who died in association with athletic exertion [18, 19, 21a, 23]. MUNSCHECK presented a similar case concerning a young sportsman of 18 [35]. On the other end of the age scale, more than 300 men of over 40 competed in the Olympic Games in Helsinki [21], while 114 men of between 60 and 84 years of age participated at the National Gymnastic Festival at Marburg in Germany in 1952 [20]. None of them came to grief as a result of their efforts. It is not likely that all of these subjects were free from coronary or myocardial lesions. Presumably, age is not a significant contributory factor in sudden death of athletes.

Clinical and Pathological Aspects

Most subjects who died suddenly in association with athletic effort and in whom autopsy revealed atherosclerotic heart disease were unaware of being afflicted with cardiac lesions [22]. Their exercise tolerance as well as their resistance to hypoxic stress [13] usually remained high until their deaths.

ZOLL [44] found that only $\frac{1}{3}$ of people with demonstrable occlusive coronary disease have angina pectoris. ENOS [9] reported that of 300 autopsies on US soldiers in their early twenties killed in action in the Korean War, 77.3% showed evidence of atherosclerotic lesions. In 20 of his cases segmental plaques reduced the lumen of a major branch of the coronaries by more than 50%. The Committee on the Effect of Strain and Trauma on Heart and Blood Vessels [37] reported in 1962 that an important degree of atherosclerosis of the coronary arteries is present in approximately 50% of all males over the age of 45 in the United States.

In 1940 GRAYBIEL [12] published the case of a 34-year-old pilot in whom a routine ECG disclosed symmetric T-Wave inversion in L 1, 2, and 4. These findings were interpreted as indicative of myocardial infarction. The evidence was considered sufficient cause to declare him unfit for flying. Since then, electrocardiographic findings of the kind under reference have generally been considered to contraindicate continued employment in hazardous occupations.

The introduction of exercise tests has added to the diagnostic relevance of electrocardiographic studies. ROBB and MARKS [38] showed that the prognosis of coronary patients whose exercise tests revealed depression of the S-T segment differed from that of patients whose exercise ECGs were normal. The coronary death rate of the former was 21 and $34^0/_{00}$ in the first and second 5-year periods following the test; that of the latter 3 and $9^0/_{00}$. On the other hand YATER et al. [42] described 4 cases of sudden cardiac death complete with autopsy findings in which normal ECGs had been obtained on the day of death, 2 days, 3 days, and 1 month before, respectively. Similarly SIMONSON [40] and DRAZIL [8] have seen several instances of sudden cardiac death of the kind under discussion verified at autopsy in subjects who had recently passed electrocardiographically monitored exercise tests. It is therefore an open question whether individuals with normal ECGs may always be granted permission to continue working in hazardous occupations. BALKE [1] reported in 1964 that the Federal Aviation Agency had recently renewed the private flying license of a pilot of 90 years of age whose clinical and electrocardiographic examination had failed to reveal signs or symptoms of cardio-vascular or other disabilities.

ROSS and LICHTLEN [39] reported that the exercise ECG may fail to indicate angiographically demonstrable obstruction of the coronary arteries. MUNSCHEK [34] found post-mortem advanced atherosclerotic coronary artery disease and a large infarct in a rower who had been medically examined 6 days prior to his death. The examination which included an ergospirometric test failed to reveal signs and symptoms indicative of the severe cardiac lesions.

Analyses of data relating to 324 cases of sudden cardiac deaths of soldiers by YATER et al. [42] showed a significantly larger number of histories of recent pneumonia and pleurisy than in a matched control group (21% as against 9%). Similarly, MEESSEN [31] who investigated the histories of and conducted autopsies on 115 soldiers who died suddenly from cardiac causes found that pulmonary infections had frequently preceded the fatal collapses. In his report of sudden non-traumatic death of soldiers DOERR [7a] emphasized that febrile infections of any kind create a situation in which strenuous physical performances may cause the death of subjects who are afflicted with a previously asymptomatic ischemic heart disease.

The majority of deaths associated with exertion occur *after* and not *during* effort. LUDES [24] has adduced evidence to the effect that in the presence of atherosclerotic coronary heart disease, a sudden drop of systolic blood pressure as is normal after physical effort may elicit an acute attack of myocardial infarction.

It is doubful whether fatal collapses of the kind under consideration are direct sequelae of myocardial ischemia even though the latter must be considered a prerequisite for the former. Restriction of the lumen of the coronary arteries through atherosclerotic deposits and plaques, progressive elimination of functioning myocardium through fibrous replacement and even the formation of thrombi such as the one seen at autopsy in the present case need not cause sudden death. Furthermore, the extent of the atherosclerotic changes in the coronary arteries of those who died in association with exercise was not always so severe as to justify their inclusion in the YATER *et al.* [43] category III ('Advanced Atherosclerosis'), as compared with categories I and II ('Early and Moderate Atherosclerosis'). Nor did our data support the unqualified validity of the suggestion made over 50 years ago by HERRICK [15] that the descending branch of the coronary artery is the 'artery of death.' Corresponding findings have been reported by other authors. FULTON [11] analyzed contrast arteriograms of hearts of individuals who had died suddenly from coronary occlusion and in whom autopsy revealed but one occluding focus. He found the descending branch of the left coronary artery involved in only 6 out of 16 cases.

No unanimity exists with regard to the significance of recent thrombi as causes of sudden death. SPAIN [41] believes that the terminal events do not necessarily depend upon the development of an acute thrombus. In a study of 568 subjects who had died from atherosclerotic coronary disease he found that the frequency of coronary thrombi increased with the length of survival from the onset of the acute fatal episode. Acute thrombi were present in only 16% of those who survived less than 1 h, but in 54% of those who survived more than 24 h. On the other hand, BÜCHNER [5] expressed the opinion that the fresh thrombus in figure 1d may well represent the immediate cause of death in the present case.

The wrestler could have lived for many more years if he had survived the syncopal attack during which he died. HELLERSTEIN [14] has described a case of spontaneous reversion of cardiac asystole after exercise in a man with hypercholesteremia, xanthomatosis, aortic stenosis, and a history of myocardial infarction who was alive 5 years following an electrocardiographically verified episode of ventricular standstill lasting 100 sec.

Physical exertion is a precipitating factor of sudden death due to myocardial ischemia like pulmonary embolism [6], *carbon monoxide poisoning* [4], *anemia* [4, 28], *low atmospheric pressure* [16, 40a], *acute blood loss* [30], and infections [19a, 2a]. Scope and magnitude of the influence of these stressors vary considerably. If several of these stressors are present at the same time, their pathogenetic effect tends to be cumulative.

Summary

Autopsy of a 45-year-old trained athlete who had died after a wrestling match revealed advanced coronary atherosclerosis and severe myocardial disease. The deceased had been free of symptoms referable to his heart; his physical performance capacity above that of most middle-aged healthy men. Exercise may be precipitating factor in sudden death of subjects with coronary heart disease. Age does not exert a predisposing influence. As to the relationship of the underlying pathological process and the terminal syncope, the evidence derived from studies of sudden cardial death of athletes suggests that myocardial ischemia, angina pectoris, coronary thrombosis, myocardial infarct and ventricular fibrillation or standstill represent pathogenic entities of their own.

References

1   BALKE, B.: Aerospace medical research and health education. Proc. Amer. Acad. Phys. Education, Dallas, Texas 1965 (cp. also AMA News, Jan. 1965).

2   BEAN, W. B.: Infarction of the heart: A morphological and clinical appraisal of 300 cases. I. Predisposing and precipitating conditions. Amer. Heart J. *14:* 684 (1937).

2 a BOURNE, G. and WEDGWOOD, J.: Heart-disease and influenza. Lancet *i:* 1226-1228 (1959).

3   BÜCHNER, F.: WEBER, A. and HAAGER, B.: Koronarinfarkt und Koronarinsuffizienz (Steinkopff, Leipzig 1935).

4   BÜCHNER, F.: Die Koronarinsuffizienz (Steinkopff, Leipzig 1939).

5   BÜCHNER, F.: Personal commun. (1965).

6   DACK, S.; MASTER, A. M.; HORN, H.; GRISHAM, A. and FIELD, L. E.: Acute coronary insufficiency due to pulmonary embolism. Amer. J. Med. *7:* 464 (1949).

7   DESANTO, D. A.: Operation and trauma as a cause of coronary and cerebral thrombosis. Amer. J. Surg. *26:* 35 (1934).

7 a DOERR, W.: Über den plötzlichen Tod aus natürlicher Ursache bei der Truppe. Wehrmed. II, pp. 109–148 (1964).

8   DRAZIL, V.: Personal commun. (1964).

9   ENOS, W. F.; HOLMES, R. H. and BEYER, J.: Coronary disease among United States soldiers killed in action in Korea (preliminary report). J. amer. med. Ass. *152:* 1090–1093 (1953).

10 FITZHUGH, G. and HAMILTON, B.: Coronary occlusion and fatal angina pectoris. J. amer. med. Ass. *100:* 475 (1933).

11 FULTON, W. F. M.: The coronary arteries (Thomas, Springfield 1965).

12 GRAYBIEL, A. and MCFARLAND, R. A.: Myocardial infarction in a young aviator. Aviat. Med. *11:* 75–80 (1940).

13 GRAYBIEL, A.: A consideration of the effects of oxygen lack of the cardiovascular system from the viewpoint of aviation. Aviat. Med. *12:* 183–190 (1941).

14 HELLERSTEIN, H. K. and TURELL, D. J.: The mode of death in coronary artery disease, an electrocardiographic and clinicopathological correlation; in Sudden cardiac death, pp. 17–37 (Grune & Stratton, New York 1964).

15 HERRICK, J. F.: Clinical features of sudden obstruction of the coronary arteries. J. amer. med. Ass. *59:* 2015 (1912).

16 HIGHMAN, B. and ALTLAND, P. D.: Acclimatisation response and pathologic changes in rats at an altitude of 25,000 feet. Arch. Path. *48:* 503 (1949).

17 JOKL, E.: Über einen spontanen Todesfall beim Sport. Schweiz. med. Wschr., *63/49:* 1278–1281 (1933).

18 JOKL, E. and MELZER, L.: Acute fatal non-traumatic collapse during work and sport. Sth afr. J. med. Sci, *5:* 4–14 (1940).

19 JOKL, E. and GREENSTEIN, J.: Fatal coronary sclerosis in a boy of ten years. Lancet *ii:* 659 (1944).

19 a JOKL, E.: Plötzlicher Sporttod durch Myokarditis bei Gonorrhoe. Haut-GeschlKr. *13:* 212–213 (1952).

20 JOKL, E.: Alter und Leistung (Springer, Berlin 1954).

21 JOKL, E.; KARVONEN, M. J.; KIHLBERG, J.; KOSKELA, A. and NORO, L.: Sports in the cultural pattern of the world. A study of the 1952 Olympic Games at Helsinki (Institute of Occupational Health, Helsinki 1956).

21 a JOKL, E.; MCCLELLAN, J. T. and ROSS, G. D.: Congenital anomaly of left coronary artery in young athlete. J. amer. med. Ass. *182:* 572–573 (1962).

22 JOKL, E.: Heart and sport (Thomas, Springfield 1964).

23 JOKL, E.: Sudden non-traumatic death associated with physical exertion, with special reference to drowning. Med. dello Sport *4:* 11–34 (1964).

24 LUDES, H. and KARSTIEN, M.: Zur Ätiologie des Herzinfarktes. Med. Welt *5:* 250–253 (1963).

25 LUTEN, D.: Contributory factors in coronary occlusion. Amer. Heart. J. *7:* 36 (1931).

26 MASTER, A. M.; DACK, S. and JAFFE, H. I.: Factors and events associated with onset of coronary thrombosis. J. amer. med. Ass. *109:* 546 (1937).

27 MASTER, A. M.; DACK, S. and JAFFE, H. L.: Premonitory symptoms of acute coronary occlusion: A study of 260 cases. Ann. intern. Med. *14:* 1155 (1941).

28 MASTER, A. M.; GUBNER, R.; DACK, S. and JAFFE, H. L.: Differentiation of acute coronary insufficiency with myocardial infarction from coronary occlusion. Arch. intern. Med. *67:* 646 (1941).

29 MASTER, A. M.: Coronary heart disease: angina pectoris, acute coronary insufficiency and coronary occlusion. Ann. intern. Med. *20:* 611 (1944).

30 MASTER, A. M.; DACK, S.; HORN, H.; FREEDMAN, B. L. and FIELD, L. E.: Acute coronary insufficiency due to acute hemorrhage: an analysis of 103 cases. Circulation, *1:* 1302 (1950).

31 MEESSEN, H.: Über den plötzlichen Herztod bei Frühsklerose und Frühthrombose. der Koronararterien bei Männern unter 45 Jahren. KreislForsch. *36:* 185 (1944)

32 MELLEROWICZ, H.: Ergometrie (Urban & Schwarzenberg, München 1962).

33 MORITZ, A. R. and ZAMCHECK, N.: Sudden and unexpected deaths of young soldiers. Arch. Path. *42:* 459–494 (1946).

34 MUNSCHECK, H.: Herztod beim Rudern infolge von arteriosklerotischem Schwielenherz. Sportarzt Sportmed. *12:* 402–409 (1962).

35 MUNSCHECK, H.: Plötzlicher Sporttod bei einem jugendlichen Boxer infolge akuter Koronarinsuffizienz, Sportarzt Sportmed. *4:* 104-111 (1964).

36 PHIPPS, C.: Contributory causes of coronary thrombosis, J. amer. med. Ass. *106:* 761 (1936).

37 Report of Committee on effect of strain and trauma on heart and great vessels. Circulation *26:* 612–622 (1962).

38 ROBB, G. P. and MARKS, H. H.: The postexercise electrocardiogram in the detection of coronary disease, a long-term evaluation. Trans. life insur. med. dir. America *45:* 81–114 (1961).

39 ROSS, R. S. and LICHTLEN, P. R., Prognostic value of coronary arteriogram; in Sudden cardiac death (Grune & Stratton, New York 1964).

40 SIMONSON, E.: Personal commun (1964).

40 a SINGH, I.; KHANNA, P. K.; HOON, R. S.; LAL, M. and RAO, B. D. P.: High-altitude pulmonary hypertension. Lancet *ii:* 146–150 (1965).

41 SPAIN, M.: Anatomical basis of sudden cardiac death; in Sudden cardiac death (Grune & Stratton, New York 1964).

42 YATER, W. M.; TRAUM, A. H.; BROWN, W. G.; FITZGERALD, R. P.; GEISLER, M. A. and WILCOX, B. B.: Coronary artery disease in men 18–39 years of age. Amer. heart J. *36:* 334–372, 481–526, 683–722 (1948).

43 YATER, W. M.; WELSH, P. P.; STAPLETON, J. F. and CLARK, M. L.: Comparison of clinical and pathologic aspects of coronary artery disease in men of various age groups: a study of 950 autopsied cases from the armed forces Institute of Pathology. Ann. intern. Med. *34:* 352–392 (1951).

44 ZOLL, P. M.: Prevention and treatment of ventricular fibrillation and ventricular asystole; in Sudden cardiac death (Grune & Stratton, New York 1964).

Authors' address: University of Kentucky, *Lexington, KY 40506* (USA)

Medicine and Sport, vol. 5: Exercise and Cardiac Death, pp. 91–98
(Karger, Basel 1971)

Congenital Anomalies of Coronary Arteries as Cause of Sudden Death Associated with Physical Exertion

J. T. McClellan and E. Jokl

A review published in 1964 of 81 cases of sudden death [4] during or shortly after physical exertion disclosed 5 instances of congenital anomalies of coronary arteries. Since then 2 additional cases have been reported [2, 6]. A resumé of the findings is submitted, preceded by a reiteration of the normal anatomy of the origin of the coronary arteries: The left coronary artery arises in the sinus of the left aortic cusp and subsequently divides into an anterior descending and a circumflex branch (fig. 1). The right coronary artery arises in the right aortic sinus and passes around the right ventricle to reach the right posterior portion of the heart. The right aortic sinus is called 'anterior sinus' according to the Basle Nomina Anatomica (BNA) nomenclature of 1895, and 'ventral sinus' according to the Jena Nomina Anatomica (NK) system of nomenclature of 1935 [6]. The nomenclature that we are using is the Internationalia Nomina Anatomica (INA) nomenclature of 1955 [6] (fig. 1).

Before describing the autopsy findings of the 7 cases of sudden death, we mention an observation whose relevance is primarily physiologic. A *post-mortem* examination was conducted on one of the best long distance runners of our time, Mr. Clarence DeMar who participated in over 1000 races, including 34 marathon competitions over 26 miles from Hopkington to Boston; of these he won 7. His last race in 1957 at the age of 68 was one of 15 km undertaken despite the presence of a colostomy necessitated by a malignant tumor which caused his death at age 70. Currens and White [3] reported that DeMar's coronary arteries were significantly large, 'estimated to be 2 or 3 times the normal diameter.' The authors commented that 'it is impossible to state whether DeMar was born with this or whether it developed as a result of long practice of great physical activity' (fig. 2a).

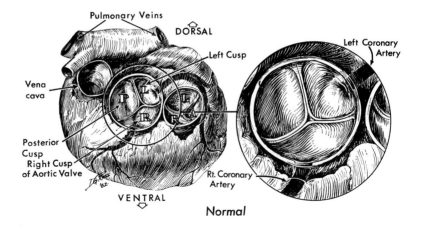

Fig. 1. The cusps of the pulmonary and aortic valves are identified in accordance with the Internationalia Nomina Anatomica (INA) approved in 1955 by the Nomenclature Committee of the International Congress of Anatomists in Paris. Textbooks of anatomy contain different references. The following table may therefore be of interest. It details the designation of the cusps of both the pulmonary and aortic valves according to the Basle Nomina Anatomica (BNA) of 1895, the Jena Nomina Anatomica (NK) laid down by the Nomenklaturkommission der Anatomischen Gesellschaft in 1935, and the INA of 1955 referred to above. The latter speaks of the pulmonary and aortic valves in their entirely as 'valvae' and of their cusps as 'valvulae'.

Valvula trunci pulmonalis	*Valvula arterii pulmonalis*	*Valva trunci pulmonalis*
A. Cuspis sinistra	A. Velum semilunare sinistrum	A. Valvula semilunaris anterior (A)
B. Cuspis dextra	B. Velum semilunare dextrum	B. Valvula semilunaris dextra (R)
C. Cuspis posterior	C. Velum semilunare dorsale	C. Valvula semilunaris sinistra (L)
Valvula aortae	*Valvula aortae*	*Valva aortae*
A. Cuspis dextra	A. Velum semilunare dextrum	A. Valvula semilunaris posterior (P)
B. Cuspis anterior	B. Velum semilunare ventrale	B. Valvula semilunaris dextra (R)
C. Cuspis sinistra	C. Velum semilunare sinistra	C. Valvula semilunaris sinistra (L)

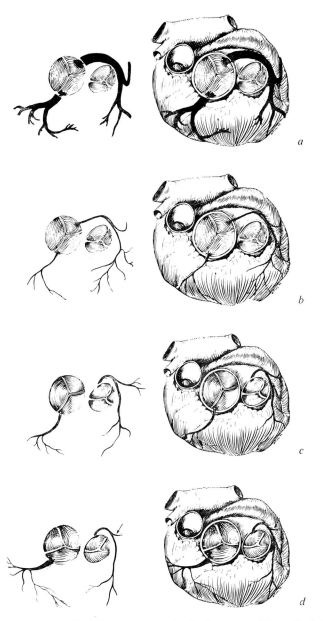

Fig. 2. Anomalies of coronary arteries in 4 cases. *a:* Generalized hypertrophy of coronary artery, *b:* generalized hypotrophy of coronary artery, *c:* left coronary artery originating from pulmonary artery, *d:* left coronary artery originating from pulmonary artery, circumflex branch withered.

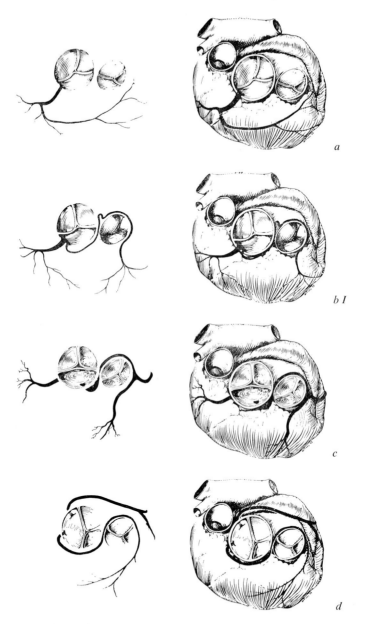

Fig. 3. Anomalies of coronary arteries in 4 additional cases. *a:* Left coronary artery absent, *b I:* both coronary arteries originating from common funnel in right aortic sinus, *c:* both coronary arteries originating separately from right aortic sinus, *d:* both coronary arteries originating from displaced right aortic cusp.

Description of Cases

The following autopsy findings of congenital abnormalities of coronary arteries appear to have been related to the deaths of the patients.

1. An internationally known rugby player, 32 years of age, collapsed after a game and died within a few minutes. His autopsy revealed a generalized hypertrophied and dilated heart weighing 482 gm. Lumina of coronary arteries and aorta were conspicuously small. The descending aorta measured ½ in in diameter, which is less than half the normal size. Microscopically several areas of myocardial fibrosis were found within the papillary muscles and at the base of the left ventricle [1] (fig. 2b).

2. A 27-year-old pneumatic drill operator died suddenly during work. The *left* coronary artery originated from the pulmonary artery. Origin and distribution of the *right* coronary artery were normal. Extensive degenerative changes were seen in the myocardium and in the papillary muscles [8] (fig. 2c).

3. A 24-year-old soldier died after a long-distance race. The *left* coronary artery originated from the pulmonary artery. The *circumflex* branch was hypoplastic, measuring only 2 cm in length. Origin and course of the *right* coronary artery were normal. Its lumen was exceptionally wide. There were diffuse multiple fibrous patches in the myocardium but no inflammatory reaction was found [7] (fig. 2d).

4. A woman, 22 years of age, who had apparently been in perfect health, died suddenly while skipping a rope after lunch. At autopsy no trace of the *left* coronary artery was found. The *right* coronary artery was of average size and the main blood supply of the left ventricle came from its descending branch. The greater part of the myocardium of the left ventricle was replaced by fibrous tissue [9] (fig. 3a).

5. A 14-year-old boy died after a cross-country race. *Both* coronary arteries originated from a common funnel in the right aortic sinus. The lumen of the *right* branch was normal, and that of the *left* was greatly reduced. There was marked hypertrophy of the left ventricle but no degenerative changes were noted in the heart muscle. The *left* coronary artery passed in the sulcus between aorta and pulmonary artery and then took a normal course, dividing into circumflex and anterior descending branches [5] (fig. 3 b I–III).

6. An 11-year-old boy collapsed after running a quarter of a mile. He was dizzy, nauseated, and soon became cyanotic; this was followed by a generalized seizure. He was admitted to a hospital. Roentgenogram of the chest suggested pulmonary edema. Death occurred 19 hours after the syncope. At *post-mortem* examination the *left* coronary artery was seen to arise behind the right aortic valve and passed between the aorta and pulmonary artery. There was a fresh infarct involving the anterolateral and the anteroseptal portions of the subendocardial portions of the myocardium. Microscopic examination revealed areas of early degenerative changes, with loss of cross-striation and infiltration with neutrophils and histiocytes. This is the only case in the series with an interval of almost 1 day between collapse and death [2] (fig. 3c).

7. A 16-year-old high school basketball player collapsed during a game and died within a few minutes. At autopsy *both* coronary arteries were seen to arise from the right sinus of the aortic valve whose cusps appeared to have been rotated clockwise around the longitudinal axis of the aorta as shown in figure 3d. A ring of connective tissue surrounded the proximal portion of the *left* coronary artery which passed through

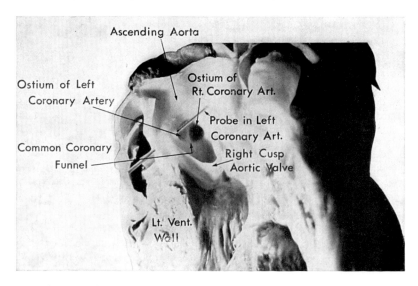

Fig. 3 b II. Two branches of coronary artery originate from common funnel above right cusp of aortic valve.

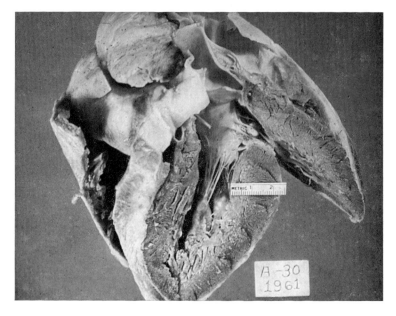

Fig. 3 b III. Marked hypertrophy of wall of left ventricle.

the sulcus between aorta and pulmonary artery. The *right* branch of the coronary artery turned dorsally and proceeded in an anteroposterior direction through the sulcus between aorta and superior vena cava. Microscopic examination failed to show pathologic changes of any kind in the coronary arteries and the myocardium [6] (fig. 3d).

Discussion

None of the cardiac anomalies under review had been identified *in vivo*. As a group the subjects were characterized by 2 clinical features: there had been no signs or symptoms indicative of the presence of heart disease, and the subjects had been able to indulge in physical activities.

Summary and Conclusions

(1) Congenital anomalies of coronary arteries may be found in individuals who die suddenly in association with physical exertion. (2) Seven subjects in whom autopsy revealed congenital anomalies of coronary arteries had been asymptomatic and able to perform physical work.

References

1   CLUVER, E. H. and JOKL, E.: Sudden death of a Rugby International after a test game. Amer. Heart J. *24:* 405–409 (1942).

2   COHEN, L. S. and SHAW, L. D.: Fatal myocardial infarction in an 11-year-old boy associated with a unique coronary artery anomaly. Amer. J. Cardiol. *19:* 420–423 (1967).

3   CURRENS, J. H. and WHITE, P. D.: Half a century of running. Clinical, physiologic, and autopsy findings in the case of Clarence DeMar ('Mr. Marathon'). New Engl. J. Med. *265:* 988 (1961).

4   JOKL, E.: Sudden non-traumatic death associated with physical exertion, with special reference to drowning. Medicina dello Sport Minerva Medica, Torino *4:* 11–34 (1964).

5   JOKL, E.; McCLELLAN, J. T., and ROSS, G. D.: Congenital anomaly of left coronary artery in young athletes. J. amer. med. Ass. *182:* 572–573 (1962).

6   JOKL, E.; McCLELLAN, J. T.; WILLIAMS, W. C.; GOUZE, F., and BARTHOLOMEW, R.: Congenital anomaly of left coronary artery in young athletes. Cardiologia *49:* 253–258 (1966).

7   PONSOLD, A.: Abgang der linken Coronararterie von der Pulmonalis als Ursache plötzlichen Todes. Dtsch. Militärarzt *4:* 137 (1939).

8   Rübberdt, H.: Abnormer Abgang der linken Kranzarterie aus der Lungenschlag-
    ader. Beitr. path. Anat. *98:* 571–578 (1937).
9   Spilsbury, B.: Death, sudden and unexpected; in Brit. Encyclopedia med. Practice,
    vol. 3, pp. 565–582 (Butterworth, London 1937).

Authors' addresses: Dr. J. T. McClellan, 1400 Harrodsburg Road, *Lexington,
KY 40504* and Prof. E. Jokl, University of Kentucky, *Lexington, KY 40506* (USA)

Medicine and Sport, vol. 5: Exercise and Cardiac Death, pp. 99–110
(Karger, Basel 1971)

Sudden Death After Exercise Due to Myocarditis

E. Jokl

After competing in a 12-mile-cross-country race in which he placed 22nd among 62 runners, a 25-year-old soldier collapsed and died. He had been known to be a good athlete, having distinguished himself over several years in gymnastic competitions.

The deceased's personal files contained a report of a medical examination conducted a few days before his death, saying that no abnormalities were detected, and that a urine examination had yielded normal results. However, it was recorded that 10 weeks earlier, he had contracted a gonorrhoic urethitis which at the time of examination was believed to have been healed.

At autopsy islands of connective tissue were scattered throughout the myocardium and histologically identified as due to sub-acute myocarditis (fig. 1 a). Interstitial infiltrates contain histiocytes and plasma cells (fig. 1 b). Hyaline degeneration of the intima caused narrowing of the caliber of the small branches of the coronary arteries only. The main branches of the coronary arteries were unaffected.

Discussion

This young athlete died in association with, but not because of, athletic exertion. Though a routine medical check a few days before the death had failed to reveal the cardiac affliction, the myocardial disease would in all probability have been identified by more thorough examination including an electrocardiographically monitored exercise test.

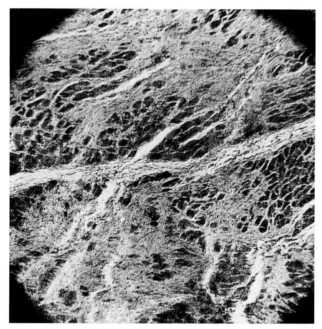

Fig. 1 a

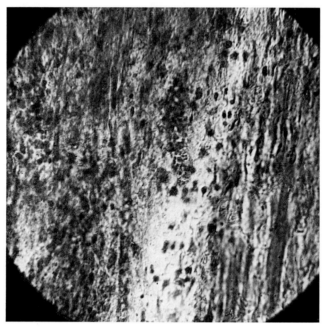

Fig. 1 b

We are impressed by the fact that in our series of autopsies on persons who died in association with exercise, the number of cases of myocarditis, acute and chronic, was much less than that of cases of coronary atherosclerosis with degenerative myocardial involvement. Before the turn of the century, KOLB[1] described the history of a champion oarsman whose competitive career was brought to an end by an attack of gonorrhoic endocarditis and myocarditis.

Reference

1   KOLB, G.: Beiträge zur Physiologie maximaler Muskelarbeit, in Gonorrhoische Endokarditis bei Meistern im Wettrudern, p. 103f (Braun, Berlin, 1898).

Authors' address: University of Kentucky, *Lexington, KY 40506* (USA)

Medicine and Sport, vol. 5: Exercise and Cardiac Death, pp. 102–111
(Karger, Basel 1971)

Sudden Death in Young Athletes

T. N. James, P. Froggatt and T. K. Marshall

Sudden unexpected death of a young athlete is not an unfamiliar event, but as part of the uniquely poignant tragedy it represents there are often few medical facts to report. In such deaths there is a limited number of possible mechanisms, of which a sudden cardiac arrhythmia is one. For this reason we have recently studied the hearts of 2 young athletes who died suddenly although previously considered to be in good health and in whom the routine necropsy provided no explanation. Special examination of the cardiac conduction system was performed in both cases, and in one it was possible to obtain a clinical and electrocardiographic survey of many surviving members of the family.

Case Histories

Patient J. W. M. (Case 1). While playing football this 18-year-old young man suddenly died. Before the game he had felt well and cycled 8 miles with his brother to the playing field. After 10 min of the match he told his brother, who was also playing, that he 'felt very tired,' and in about 30 sec he collapsed. Only a few minutes later, on admission to the local rural hospital located beside the football ground, he was dead.

Further history was obtained from his parents and family. The only possible teratogenic factor unearthed was a febrile illness that kept his mother in bed for about 2 weeks during the 4th or 5th month of pregnancy. His childhood was spent in good health until the age of 13, when he began to complain of tiredness, headache, loss of appetite, and difficulty in sleeping. His doctor then noticed a slow irregular pulse for which the boy was referred for outpatient consultation in a small rural hospital. There the pulse was described as 58/min and 'irregular,' and an apical systolic murmur was noted; a chest X ray was negative, but an electrocardiogram (EKG) was not done. At the age of 14 he was again seen in consultation, but again no EKG was made: At rest the pulse was about 42/min with coupled beats; on exercise it sped up to 70/min and was regular without coupling. A systolic murmur in the pulmonic area was now described, but the examiner felt that the symptoms were mainly of emotional origin. A sedative was prescribed, and he was referred to a child guidance clinic.

About 2½ years before death he was working as message boy on a bicycle when he was found one day disoriented with occipital abrasions. It was assumed that his head injury was caused by falling off his bicycle, but this was never established. At the hospital he said that he had caught his foot on the pedal and must have fallen and hit his head, but his father suggested that the boy had 'blacked out' first. He was probably unconscious for a short period. At an examination 1 h later, the pulse was 80 min and regular, and a skull X ray was negative. He was discharged after 3 days. There is no clear history of any subsequent episodes of loss of consciousness or orientation, although they cannot be entirely ruled out since he would never discuss his health with anyone, even his family. They thought he worried about something all the time, but the object is not known.

Family history: Both parents are members of huge sibships. There is no history of relevant or suspicious symptoms in the members traced except as noted below. Specifically, there is no history of sudden unexpected death, deafness, epileptoid seizures, breath-holding episodes, respiratory distress syndrome, heart condition, or consanguinity. The propositus had 2 sisters and 1 brother. The brother and 1 sister were asymptomatic and had normal EKGs; the other sister has been extremely apprehensive about her heart since her brother's death and complains of palpitation and indigestion. She is considered a nervous woman. Her physical examination and EKG were normal except for premature beats of supraventricular origin. The two children of this sister are normal. Information is available about 75 uncles, aunts, and cousins of the propositus and is pertinent in only 2. A maternal aunt had blackouts before a hysterectomy for menorrhagia some years ago, presumably due to anemia since they stopped after the operation; examination included an EKG and was normal. A male first cousin, aged 12 years, is the son of the maternal aunt and was well until he fainted while watching television one evening; his EKG is normal (rather prominent U waves in V_2 and V_3), but an EEG was interpreted to show 'well-marked epileptic response to photic stimulation over a wide range of flash rates.'

Both parents are 58 years old, have no complaints pertinent to the case, and have essentially normal physical examinations. EKGs were made on each parent on 2 occasions 6 months apart. On both occasions that of the father was within normal limits, with a PR interval of about 0.21 sec. In the first tracing of the mother there were repeated episodes of transient sinus arrest, but these were not present on the second examination; other features of the EKG were normal.

Necropsy findings: Only the heart was abnormal. The coronary arteries, pericardium, cardiac valves and septa, and myocardial thickness and architecture were all normal. The arteries supplying both the atrioventricular (AV) node and the sinus node originated from the right coronary artery at the usual sites [1–3]. Gross examination of the conduction system was normal except for some ecchymoses near the posterior margin of the sinus node. The area of sinus node was originally screened with sections from 17 serial blocks each about 2 mm thick and that of the AV node and the His bundle, from 10 similar blocks. In regions requiring additional examination serial 6-μ sections were subsequently made from the original blocks so that a total of 85 slides were studied. The ventricular myocardium was histologically normal, and the significant histopathology was in and near the conduction system.

The most striking changes were in the sinus node. For a distance of several milli-meters the sinus node artery was markedly narrowed by a bizarre medial hyperplasia, and at several points the pinhole lumen was completely occluded by additional intimal proliferation (fig. 1 and 2). This change in the sinus node artery is identical to that observed in a variety of diseases in which arrhythmias have been documented (4–9). There were foci of both old (scars) and recent (hemorrhage and degeneration) injury within the sinus node and its adjacent nerves and ganglia (fig. 3). Minor changes in the AV node and the His bundle consisted of a small amount of intimal proliferation in one branch of the AV mode artery with moderate narrowing of its lumen and unusually heavy deposits of collagen partitioning portions of both the AV node and the His bundle. Slips of AV nodal fibers extend into the central fibrous body in blind pockets, and a few of these fibers were degenerating without inflammatory reaction. A tiny degenerative focus no more than a few microns across was present in part of the left bundle branch.

Patient A. C. (case 2). On an autumn afternoon this 15-year-old boy was playing with 5 companions on some grassy waste ground. They had formed 2 teams of 3 each and were wrestling, the object being to hold an opponent down on his back. They had been playing for 10 or 15 min during which time this boy had occasionally somersaulted forward and at least once had stood on his head. There was a bank of clay soil dumped by contractors who were digging foundations near by, and this contained some stones and a few bricks. At one stage he fell on this bank and rolled down the slope to the foot. When he got up he was clasping his left side, but after a few seconds he carried on playing again. Three minutes later he sat down in the field and said that he felt sick. Then he lay down on his back and turned blue. He did not speak after that, and the boys called 2 men. One tried artificial respiration, and the other sent for an ambulance. He was un-conscious but still alive when the ambulance left for the hospital but was dead on arrival there 17 min after first complaining of feeling sick.

These events were in midafternoon. After his lunch he had bought some apples from mobile shop, and it is thought that he had eaten more than one of these on his way down to the waste ground. All considered him in good health, and he had recently been working as a lorry helper. At the age of 8 years he had an operation for a depressed fracture of the skull, and when 13 years old he received treatment of a rupture. He last saw a doctor 9 months before death because of a septic throat. He was one of a large family (10 or 11 siblings), and there is apparently no history of untoward attacks, although efforts to obtain more specific information from the family have been unsuccessful.

Necropsy findings: The case initially appeared as one of natural death, but an intra-abdominal injury due to the fall needed to be excluded, as did choking and laryngeal shock due to aspiration of food, although the latter seemed unlikely in view of his speaking after feeling ill. At necropsy there was no internal injury. There was 1 oz of straw-colored fluid in each pleural cavity, some regurgitated food just above the vocal cords and a few particles in the trachea, a slight excess of yellow watery fluid in the abdominal cavity, and nothing else. *A few necrotic muscle fibers* with round-cell infiltration were observed widely scattered in 4 of 13 representative sections of *left ventricular myocardium,* and there was a small amount of nonspecific *perivascular fibrosis* with occasional *focal medial degeneration in small coronary arteries and arterioles.* In the lungs there were some conges-tion and edema with a few patches of aspiration autolysis. None of these findings was considered an adequate explanation for his sudden unexpected death, and attention was then concentrated on the cardiac conduction system.

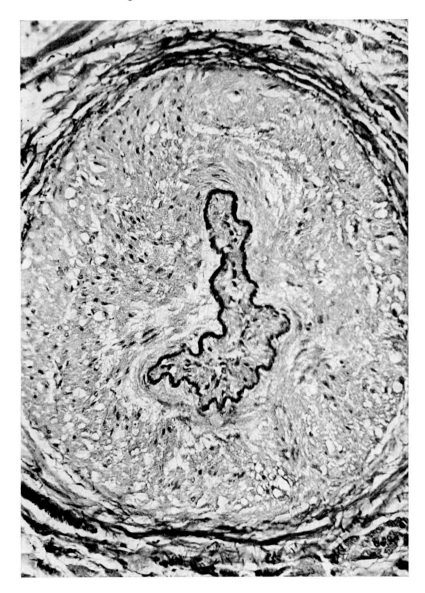

Fig. 1. Branch of sinus node artery of patient in case 1. Verhoeff-van Gieson stain, × **300**.

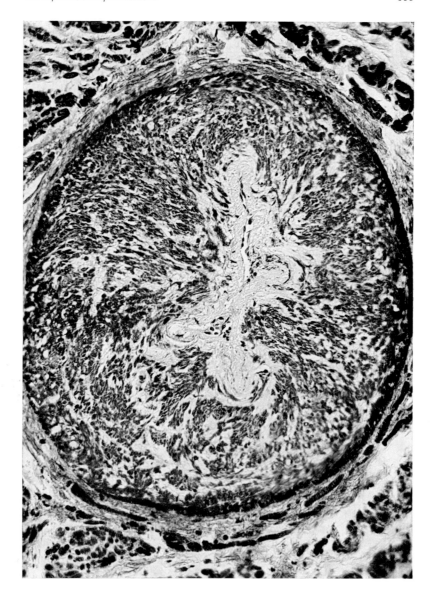

Fig. 2. Section from same artery, Goldner trichrome stain, × 300.

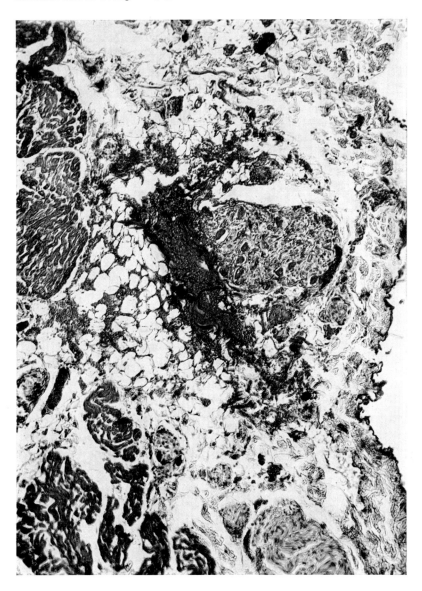

Fig. 3. Hemorrhage adjacent to ganglion near the sinus node (case 1). Goldner trichrome stain, × 140.

Except as noted above, cardiac findings outside the conduction system were not remarkable. The regions of sinus node, AV node, and His bundle were prepared in a manner similar to that for case 1, with a total of 198 sections being studied. A number of microscopic *foci of degeneration* were present in the *AV* node and the *His bundle*, but all but one these were *old scarring*; the exception was an area approximately 100 μm across at the posterior margin of the AV node where there was *recent necrosis with round-cell infiltration*. As in the first case, however, the more impressive pathology was in the *sinus node*. The main sinus node artery was thickened, but one of its major branches supplying nutrient circulation to the node was nearly occluded by medial hyperplasia and intimal proliferation. Downstream from this point of occlusion there was a relatively large focus of degeneration in the sinus node, including a number of adjacent nerves and ganglia.

Discussion

There is a saddening paradox in the sudden death of a young athlete, representing as it does the abrupt end of vigor, strength, and youth, qualities that seem the essence of continuing life. Partly because of the unavoidable personal feelings stirred by such death there has been growing recent interest in the problem, out of proportion to its numerical frequency among all deaths. High school football deaths are a notable example, where any may be rightfully considered too many. Those interested in sports medicine have constantly improved protective equipment to prevent dangerous injuries and have continually revised game rules to reduce accidents. Despite these efforts, however, a number of sudden deaths in games remain unexplained, and it is relative to these that the present observations have particular pertinence.

The findings are best interpreted as compatible with a terminal cardiac arrhythmia, but the prevalence of changes in the sinus node raises some questions as to how a lethal arhythmia may have developed. It must be conceded that the lesser magnitude of histopathologic changes in the atrioventricular (AV) node and the His bundle does not necessarily mean lesser functional significance, and it is not difficult to understand how abrupt heart block, for example, may be fatal. Prudence suggests that the grosser pathology be considered most carefully, however, particularly when it was not only similar in both cases but also resembled that observed in a number of other diseases associated with sudden death [4–9].

Among deaf children with spells who die suddenly a very similar lesion has been observed in the sinus node [8, 9], and the same question arose as to how such a lesion could be fatal. In the deaf children 2 factors were considered. The 1st was the presence of a prolonged QT interval (characteristic of the syndrome), causing increased duration of the ventricular vulnerable period, during which a critically timed atrial premature beat or even atrial fibrillation may lead to a ventricular arrhythmia [10, 11]. On the basis of this reasoning it was predicted that continued observations in deaf children with long QT intervals and syncopal attacks should lead to documentation of paroxysms of ventricular arrhythmia [8, 12], and these have now been reported by several observers [13–15]. Unfortunately, neither of the 2 young athletes had had an EKG. Among the family of one an electrocardiographic survey was conducted partly to look for QT prolongation, which is a heritable trait, and a search was made for the congenital deafness that is often (but not always) associated. No significant QT prolongation was found, but this does not eliminate its possible presence in either of the deceased. Furthermore, even those with significant QT prolongation do not always show this change on serial study.

The other factor among the deaf children with injuries in the sinus node that was considered contributory to the development of a lethal cardiac arrhythmia was hemorrhage and degeneration in the regions of juxtanodal nerves and ganglia. If these led to neuroflexes, those originating in the ganglia (and some of the nerves) must be vagal since it is generally thought that there are no adrenergic ganglia in the heart. Cholinergic reflexes at the time of intracardiac neural ischemia must suppress sinus pacemaking and AV conduction and may simultaneously suppress the ability of other efficient pacemaking sites (such as the AV node or the His bundle) to provide an efficient escape rhythm. Thus, the occluded sinus node artery might not only alter function of the sinus node directly but by leading to vagal discharge might further depress sinus and other efficient mechanisms as well as impair AV conduction.

Among the kindred of Patient I a significant abnormality was present in the EKG of his mother on one occasion but not later. This was intermittent sinus arrest, which has also been observed in some deaf children and their kindred [9]. This, as well as other disorders of normal sinus pacemaking, would actually be the type of functional abnormality one might anticipate with sinus nodal ischemia. Of further significance in this regard is the clear record of marked bradycardia in the first case, which may also be interpreted as a form of abnormal function of the sinus node, whether the actual rhythm during the slow heart rate was sinus bradycardia or sinus arrest with an escape bradycardia of ectopic origin.

Recent studies by HAN, DeTRAGLIA, MILLET, *and* MOE [16] *have demonstrated that a slow heart rate itself produces conditions favorable to the development of ectopic beats and fibrillation because of the greater range of refractory periods at various points in the ventricles.*

It has long been known that well-trained athletes characteristically have a slow heart rate. A number of studies have been conducted to determine the physiologic mechanism of this observation, which is at least partly dependent on a high level of vagal tone. Neither of the subjects of the present study could properly be considered a highly trained athlete, but the findings in their hearts may be important relative to those athletes with extensive training. If the training process does produce a vagal effect, one manifestation of which is sinus bradycardia, then the additional presence of disease in the sinus node may be compounded, and it may be the latter that is the lethal factor in those athletes who die suddenly and unexpectedly. This should be relatively simple to determine by examining the cardiac conduction system in such fatal cases, an investigation that has not previously been done to our knowledge.

But easily the most important practical point of the present observations is the probability that under ideal conditions both boys could have been resuscitated. Conditions during athletic games are not always ideal, particularly in rural and other isolated areas, but a number of sudden deaths in young athletes have occurred within a short distance of medical facilities for emergency resuscitation. Undoubtedly some physicians with a special interest in sports medicine have considered the possibility of an arrhythmia as the lethal event in sudden deaths, but it is probably accurate to say that many have not. The findings in these 2 young athletes indicate that this possibility must be promptly considered, in addition to the more obvious extracardiac injuries, whenever a young athlete collapses suddenly. In both these cases the general myocardium was well preserved, and with normal electrical activity it should have supported not only life but continued vigor.

Summary

The sudden unexpected deaths of 2 young athletes and the findings in their hearts at necropsy are described. Based on the histopathology in and around the sinus node, which was the same in both hearts, a terminal cardiac arrhythmia is postulated as the mechanism of death. Ways in which ischemic pathology in and near the normal cardiac pacemaker may lead to a lethal arrhythmia are discussed. Stress is placed on the importance of considering a cardiac arrhythmia when examining athletes who have suddenly collapsed, since the present observations indicate that appropriate treatment should produce complete recovery.

References

1   JAMES, T. N.: *Anatomy of the coronary arteries.* Hoeber Medical Division, New York (1961).

2   JAMES, T. N.: Anatomy of the human sinus node. *Anat. Rec. 141:* 109 (1961).

3   JAMES, T. N.: Morphology of the human atrioventricular node, with remarks pertinent to its electrophysiology. *Amer. Heart J. 62:* 756 (1961).

4   JAMES, T. N.: Observations on the cardiovascular involvement, including the cardiac conduction system, in progressive muscular dystrophy. *Amer. Heart. J. 63:* 48 (1962).

5   JAMES, T. N. and FISCH, C.: Observations on the cardiovascular involvement in Friedreich's ataxia. *Amer. Heart J. 66:* 164 (1963).

6   JAMES, T. N.; FRAME, B. and SCHATZ, I. J.: Pathology of the cardiac conduction system in Marfan's syndrome. *Arch. intern. Med. 114:* 339 (1961).

7   JAMES, T. N.: An etiologic concept concerning the obscure myocardiopathies. *Prog. cardiovasc. Dis., 7:* 48 (1964).

8   FRASER, G. R.; FROGGATT, P. and JAMES, T. N.: Congenital deafness associated with electrocardiographic abnormalities, fainting attacks and sudden death. A recessive syndrome. *Quart. J. Med. 33:* 361 (1964).

9   JAMES, T. N.: Congenital deafness and cardiac arrhythmias. *Amer. J. Cardiol. 19:* 627 (1967).

10 PRESTON, J. B.; McFADDEN, S. and MOE, G. K.: Atrioventricular transmission in young mammals. *Amer. J. Physiol. 197:* 236 (1959).

11 MOORE, E. N.: Microelectrode studies on concealment of multiple premature atrial responses. *Circ. Res. 18:* 660 (1966).

12 Annotation: Congenital cardiac arrhytmia. *Lancet ii:* 26 (1964).

13 BARLOW, J. B.; BOSMAN, C. K. and COCHRANE, J. W. C.: Congenital cardiac arrhythmia (letter to the editor). Lancet *ii:* 531 (1964).

14 GAMSTORP, I.; NILSEN, R. and WESTLING, H.: Congenital cardiac arrhythmia. Lancet *ii:* 965 (1964).

15 WARD, O. C.: A new familial cardiac syndrome in children. *J. ir. med. As. 54:* 103 (1964).

16 HAN, J.; DeTRAGLIA, J.; MILLET, D. and MOE, G. K.: Incidence of ectopic beats as a function of basic rate in the ventricle. *Amer. Heart J. 72:* 632 (1966).

For reprints: Dr. T. N. JAMES, University of Alabama, Medical Center, *Birmingham, AL 35233* (USA)

Medicine and Sport, vol. 5: Exercise and Cardiac Death, pp. 112–120
(Karger, Basel 1971)

Deaths from Exposure on Four Inns Walking Competition, March 14–15, 1964 [1]

L. G. C. E. Pugh

Organisation

The Four Inns walking competition has been held annually for the last 7 years and is organised by the 51st Derby (St. Luke's) California Rover Crew. It is very popular in the Scouting movement. This year 80 three-man teams started; a further 40 teams applied to enter but were turned down for lack of accommodation. The age-range of the participants is from 17½ to 24 years. There are both team and individual trophies. The course involves a 45-mile walk over the moors at altitudes ranging from 650 ft to 2000 ft and a total ascent and descent of about 4500 ft. The record time is 7½ h. However, competitors usually take from 9½ to 22 h. I understand that up to ⅓ of the competitors give up, most of them after the toughest sections, either at Snake Inn (16 miles) or Edale (24 miles). There have been cases of fatigue but no accidents or fatalities.

Precautions

Preliminary and final information sheets are circulated which contain details of the course, the system of tallies, the kit required, and so on. A pamphlet containing advice about clothing is also issued. There are

---

1   This report is based on evidence heard at the inquest held at Glossop on April 8, and on the written reports of members of the Glossop District Rover Crew Mountain Rescue Team.

check-points at intervals of 3 to 8 miles along the route and a rescue team is on call. From reading the information sheets it is clear that the organisers have taken great care to safeguard the participants. They also follow the weather forecasts for several days before the race. The reason given for holding the competition so early in the year is that March is the most convenient month from the point of view of school and university examinations.

The 1964 Event

The 80 three-man teams started at 2-min intervals beginning at 6 a.m. The weather forecast that morning was that there would be showers with fine intervals. Actually there was drizzle and a light wind at the start, and the weather deteriorated all day with heavy rain and strong winds. During the night there was sleet and snow (from 4.30 a.m.). Temperatures recorded by 4 meteorological stations in the area (supplied by the Meteorological Office) ranged between 4°C and 7°C during the day with a night minimum of 3°C on March 14–15. Temperatures on the moors at 2000 ft would be about 3°C lower than these readings. Winds near sea-level were up to 25 knots in velocity, but were probably much stronger on the moors.

Of the 240 competitors only 90 were competing for the first time. This year only 22 competitors finished. Usually only ⅓ drop out: one year 85% finished.

At about 1.15 p.m. the check-point at Snake Inn, about 16 miles from the start, received word that some competitors were in difficulties, and the Glossop Mountain Rescue Team began rescue operations. (The section before Snake Inn is the most difficult part of the route and contains a long ascent of 1300 ft over boggy ground.) They brought down 5 exhausted walkers (2 in a state of collapse) and escorted a number of others who had retired. They got to Gordon Withers at about 2 p.m. He was then conscious and able to walk with assistance, but he later collapsed and was transported on a stretcher. The rescue took 5 h altogether.

Later in the afternoon a search was started for 2 competitors who were stated to be sheltering about 4½ mile off course near the River Alport. The rescuers never made contact with these men, and their bodies were found 2 days later. Witnesses at the inquest said that the weather conditions were severe but they were accustomed to such conditions, although not for so long.

Over 800 persons took part in the 2-day search for the missing competitors, i.e. Welby and Butterfield.

Case Histories

G. Withers. Student. Aged 19. 11 years a Scout; took part in the Four Inns Walk in 1962 and 1963. Severe attack of influenza 3 weeks previously.

According to his team-mates, Withers began to flag around midday after the long climb to Bleaklow (2000 ft) which they all found very tiring. By this time had been out some $5\frac{1}{2}$ h and had covered about 12 miles. They were wet and cold. Withers began to fall down frequently and his companions had to walk one on each side of him. Shortly afterwards, they sat down and one of them went for help, which arrived within 2 h. Withers was then conscious and able to walk with assistance. At about 4.15 p.m. rescuer Dean stated that he was semiconscious and incoherent. By this time he was being carried by 3 rescuers. While they were carrying him along a narrow steep slope he had a convulsion which threw the rescuers off their balance, and one of them fell 20 ft and hurt his chest. Eventually they were met by a stretcher party, and Withers was carried on the stretcher in a thick kapok sleeping-bag with waterproof cover. It was reported that on arrival at Alport Farm at 7.15 p.m., Withers' body was rigid and he had become very pale. A pulse was detectable at his temple. It was not stated whether he was conscious or not. 1 h later, at 8.15 p.m., he was admitted to Glossop Hospital apparently dead. Artificial respiration and oxygen were given for 3 h without success.

Necropsy. Average build, abrasions of knees and wrists. Lungs, liver, and kidneys congested. Heart enlarged and congested; right ventricle distended and wall 'thinned out'. Cause of death: acute myocardial failure after extreme exposure to cold. The pathologist thought that the attack of influenza might have contributed.

J. Butterfield and M. Welby. Students, both aged 21, and members of the same team. They were experienced hikers and Welby had taken part in the Four Inns Walk in 1962. The 3rd member of the team was R. Kydd, aged 19, and he gave evidence at the inquest.

The team started at 7.45 a.m. Near Bleaklow, Butterfield complained of cramp and kept stopping. He was going more and more slowly. They were all very wet; at this stage they lost their way and went about 1 mile off course. The time was not stated but it was probably early afternoon. Butterfield became unsteady and his companions had to urge him on. In the words of Kydd, 'Butterfield was slowly tiring and getting unsteady. We had to help him although I was not much good because I was stumbling too.' They helped him by walking on each side. He did not say much, but when he did speak his voice was normal. When he could go no further they sat down, and Welby, who was the fittest, went to reconnoitre. When he returned, Kydd went to fetch help while Welby stayed with Butterfield. Kydd met a rescue party and was assisted down to Alport Farm, suffering from exposure. Two parties searched for Welby and Butterfield but failed to find them.

It is thought Welby may have stayed with Butterfield until he died, and started back perhaps in the dark, when his torch may have given out. Their bodies were found 2 days later. Butterfield's body was in a stream bed, partly in the water. Welby's body was lying covered with snow about 1 mile to the west.

Necropsy. The findings were essentially similar to the findings on Withers, except that the organs were less congested.

D. Read. Sometime between 3.30 p.m. and 4 p.m. this competitor was found sheltering under the wall of a sheep pen. Rescuer Davies stated he was semiconscious. He was carried down on a stretcher to Snake Inn and later admitted to Glossop Hospital where he recovered.

R. Kydd. Kydd was the 3rd member of the team to which Butterfield and Welby belonged. When Rescuer Simm met him on the way to the Snake Inn he was exhausted. To quote Rescuer Simm: 'He was able to inform me that he had to leave 2 of his team mates up the valley...but due to his condition he could not give me the exact location.' Kydd was accompanied down to the Snake Inn by 2 rescuers. There he recovered, and later he was transported to Buxton base camp.

Comments

Weather. Weather conditions were severe but not exceptional. The official forecast was wrong. Temperatures on the moors would have between +1°C and +4°C, which, in the presence of strong winds and rain, is a typical wet-cold situation. It would clearly be safer to postpone the annual race until later in the season when the weather is warmer and the days longer.

Clothing. The clothing of the dead boys was produced in court. Each outfit consisted of (1) an anorak: 2 were of poor quality and 1 satisfactory; (2) a jersey: one light-weight, others medium; (3) a shirt and singlet; (4) trousers: 1 jeans, 1 33% terylene-wool mixture; 1 corduroy; (5) socks: 2–3 pairs each; (6) climbing boots: of good quality.

The trousers afforded little protection against wind and rain. Anoraks, however good, will not keep a man dry for more than 2–3 h; for, to avoid condensation, they have to be made of permeable cloth. Witnesses did not seem to appreciate this. All competitors who gave evidence said they were wet through and very cold. A patrol warden for the Peaks National Park said he always wore an oilskin on the moors in wet weather.

Public attention needs to be called to the dangers of the wet-cold environment. These boys would have been all right if they not been wet through. They were lightly clad because it was a race. The organisers might consider making it compulsory to carry spare clothing and a plastic rain-proof coat.

Food. All the witnesses said they had enough food with them in the form of chocolate and raisins, and coffee and soup was issued at the check-points. I should not expect a calorie intake of more than 1000–1500 kcal. on an exercise of this kind, although the total energy expenditure may be over 6000 kcal.

Heat balance. The oxygen consumption of men walking in mountains at a pace they can maintain over many hours has been measured in various parts of the world and is generally about 2·0 l/min for a 75-kg man in good training (table 1). The record-holders on the Four Inns Walk have been long-distance runners, and can probably maintain an oxygen consumption of a least 3·0 l/min. For the average competitor a figure of 1·5–2·0 l is likely. The corresponding heat production values are 900 kcal/h and 450–600 kcal/h.

These values are similar to the values observed in cross-Channel swimming races. Channel swimming is in some respects similar to hill walking in that it involves a high rate of energy expenditure over a very long period. Some years ago it was found [PUGH and EDHOLM, 1955; PUGH *et al.*, 1960] that fast swimmers maintained *normal rectal temperatures* after 9–10 h in water at 15ºC, although they were relatively thin. Slow swimmers became hypothermic unless they were fat. Fast relatively thin swimmers became hypothermic if they got tired and slowed down. In hill walking under conditions of wet-cold the situation may be much the same. The stronger teams who can maintain a fast pace produce

Table I. Determination of oxygen intake and heat production in 8 subjects during steady prolonged climbing at the subject's habitual place.

Subject	Altitude	Oxygen consumption (l/min)	Heat production (kcal/h)	Locality
G. P.	1000	1·88	565	North Wales
G. P.	3500	2·00	600	Swiss Alps
G. P.	6000	2·18	654	Himalaya
M. W.	6000	1·89	567	Himalaya
A. S.	2000	2·32	700	Scotland
J. B.	2000	2·53	757	Scotland
J. B.	2000	2·03	608	Scotland
M. W.	2000	2·30	689	Scotland
Mean		2·14	641	—

Adjusted to equal body-weight of 75 kg (165 lb) [DURNIN, 1955; PUGH, 1958].

heat at a high enough rate to keep themselves warm in spite of the low insulation value of wet clothing. Slower walkers, or fast walkers slowed down by fatigue, may not have a high enough heat production for thermal equilibrium, in which case they will cool slowly over a period of hours until a state is reached where balance and muscular control are impaired. At this stage their pace begins to fall off, and owing to the associated decline in heat production, the rate of body cooling may be expected to accelerate.

According to the above case-histories, the onset of collapse follows within 1–2 h after a person begins to slow down. Once serious body cooling has occurred, warming by natural means takes many hours. In the case of Withers, the kapok sleeping-bag and cover used by the rescuers were ineffective. On the other hand, if a man is only moderately impaired, whether by fatigue or cold, he may recover rapidly with rest in a warm environment.

Signs and symptoms. In these cases the signs of impairment, whether through cold or fatigue, were slowing (followed by clumsiness and stumbling), falling, and finally collapse. Mental symptoms were not apparent until a late stage.

Table II. Theoretical estimate of minimum insulation value of clothing worn on Four Inns walking competition, when wet through.

Heat production	500 kcal/h
Body-surface area	2.0 m²
Body-weight	75 kg
Heat production/m² body surface (M)	250 kcal., h^{-1}
Evaporative heat loss (E) from lungs and skin at 20% of M	50 kcal., h^{-1}
Heat loss through clothing and exposed skin (H)	200 kcal., m^{-2}, h^{-1}
Ambient air temperature (t_a)	+2°C
Mean skin temperature (t_s)	30°C
Thermal gradient $t_s — t_a$	28
Total insulation, i.e. clothing (I_{cl}) and air (I_a)	$\dfrac{28}{200} = \dfrac{0.14°C}{kcal., m^{-2}, h^{-1}}$ $= 0.78$ clo units

The insulation value of the surrounding air in winds of 25-knot velocity and over is nearly constant at around 0·1 clo unit [BURTON and EDHOLM, 1955]. Hence the insulation value of the average competitor's clothing on the Four Inns Competition in wet stormy weather at temperature of 2°C would be 0·78—0·1 = 0·68 clo unit. When dry the same outfit would have an insulation value of not less than 1·5 clo units.

Clothing insulation. The clothing worn by the dead boys was brought back to Hampstead. The thermal insulation of the 3 sets of clothes, both wet and dry, will be determined in our climatic chamber. Meanwhile it is possible to make an approximate assessment, based on certain assumptions (tables 1 and 2). Inspection of the clothing suggests a value of about 1·5 clo units for the dry state.[2] If one assumes a mean rate of heat production of 500 kcal/h, the minimum clothing insulation for thermal balance works out at 0·68 clo units. This seems a likely value for the clothing when wet through. It would mean that competitors unable to maintain a heat production of 500 kcal/h would gradually cool down, whereas in dry clothing they could just keep warm with a heat production of 330 kcal/h. This is equivalent to an oxygen consumption of 1·1 l/min, which is the oxygen consumption required for walking on level ground at 3 miles an hour.

The calculations are as follows (symbols as in table 2):

The minimum heat production for warmth with dry clothing is 1·5 clo (table II). Let

$$I_a + I_{cl} = 1\cdot5 + 0\cdot1 = 1\cdot6 \text{ clo} = 1\cdot6 \times 0\cdot18 = 0\cdot288 \ \frac{^{o}C}{kcal.} \ m^{-2}, h^{-1}.$$

For warmth, t_s will be not less than 32·5°C and

$$t_s - t_a = 30.5°C.$$

Hence heat loss through clothing and exposed skin (H) is

$$\frac{30\cdot5}{0\cdot288} = 106 \text{ kcal., } m^{-2}, h^{-1}$$

and $M = H + E = 106 + 50 = 165$ kcal., m^{-2}, h^{-1}.

Hence metabolism for a 75-kg man is 330 kcal/h, and oxygen consumption is

$$\frac{330}{300} = 1\cdot1 \text{ l/min.}$$

This is the oxygen requirement for level walking at 3 m/h.

Conclusions and Suggested Recommendations

1. The risk of casualties from exposure could be avoided by holding the competition later in the year, when the weather is warmer and the days are longer.

2. Competitors should not be allowed to start unless they are carrying spare clothing, a plastic mackintosh (or other waterproof outer garment)

2   1 clo unit is the amount of insulation required for thermal equilibrium in an environment of 21°C (70°F) with minimal air movement and 50% humidity. This is the insulation afforded by the clothing worn in summer by the average business man. 1 clo = 0·18°C/kcal., m^{-2}, h^{-1}.

and waterproof trousers (i.e., plastic impregnated nylon as used in sailing: price about 40*s*.).

3. Anoraks have to be made of permeable materials to avoid condensation. Chemical proofing and fine weave gives partial protection against wetting but no anorak can be expected to keep a man dry all day. Jeans, or trousers of terylene-wool mixture, are neither windproof nor waterproof, and are unsuitable at temperatures near freezing-point in the presence of strong winds, except for walks of less than 2–3 hours' duration.

4. In view of the relatively short period between the onset of symptoms and collapse, early symptoms such as slowing and incoordination call for urgent action (dry clothing; shelter; get off the mountain).

5. As long as a man can walk, evacuation is quick. Once he is a stretcher case it is dangerously slow.

6. In view of (5) methods of on-the-spot resuscitation of stretcher cases require urgent development.

Summary

1. The 8th Annual Four Inns Walking Competition (45 miles) took place in wet-cold conditions, the air temperatures on the moors being 2–3°C. There was heavy rain most of the day, and a strong wind. The official weather report was misleading.

2. From the 5th hour some competitors began to get into difficulties. Three Scouts lost their lives and at least 4 others had narrow escapes.

3. The clothing of the dead men was not waterproof, and the trousers were not windproof.

4. The cause of death was given as exposure to prolonged cold. In 1 of 3 cases a severe attack of influenza 3 weeks previously was thought to have been contributory. There were no significant necropsy findings other than terminal congestion.

5. Symptoms of exposure, in order of development, were: (a) slowing of the rate of progress, clumsiness, and stumbling; (b) repeated falling; (c) inability to continue; (d) incoherence, impairment of consciousness; (e) unconsciousness, extreme pallor, and in one case what appears to have been a convulsion. In these cases mental symptoms were late in appearance.

6. Only about 2 h elapsed between first symptoms and collapse.

7. Evacuation of one of the fatal cases took 5 h.

8. Mild cases recovered with rest and warmth.

9. The race was well organised and all recognised safety precautions were taken.

References

BURTON, A. C., EDHOLM, O. G.: Man in a cold environment; p. 50 (Edward Arnold, London 1955).
DURNIN, J. V. G. A. J. Physiol. *128:* 294 (1955).
PUGH, L. G. C.: J. Physiol. *141:* 233 (1958).
PUGH, L. G. C. and EDHOLM, O. G.: Lancet *ii:* 761 (1955).
PUGH, L. G. C.; EDHOLM, O. G.; FOX, R. H.; WOLFF, H. S.; HARVEY, G. R.; HAMMOND, W. H.; TANNER, J. M., and WHITEHOUSE, R. H.: Clin. Sci. *19:* 257 (1960).

Author's address: Dr. L. G. C. E. PUGH, Division of Human Physiology, National Institute for Medical Research, Holly Hill, *London N. W. 3* (England)

Medicine and Sport, vol. 5: Exercise and Cardiac Death, pp. 121-147
(Karger, Basel 1971)

Nephropathy Associated with Heat Stress and Exercise

R. W. Schrier, H. S. Henderson, C. C. Tisher and R. L. Tannen

Heat stress and exercise may result in severe medical consequences in both military and civilian populations. In World War I, Willcox [1] reported 462 heatstroke deaths in 1 month among British Expeditionary Forces arriving in Mesopotamia. Though on a much smaller scale in World War II, British troops in Iraq again suffered significant heat casualties [2]. In a *post-mortem* study, Malamud, Haymaker and Custer [3] selected 125 fatal cases of heatstroke that occurred in the United States military training installations during World War II.

Several epidemics of heat illness in civilian populations have occurred in the United States [4–7]. Gauss and Meyer [4] stated that the majority of their 158 heatstroke patients were manual laborers, and others were firemen, cooks, and laundry workers. Other occupations as well as religious practices have also been predisposing factors. A significant incidence of heat illness has been cited on oil tankers in the Persian Gulf [8] and in African gold mines [9]. During the Mecca Pilgrimages from 1959 to 1961 there were 1,025 deaths related to heat illness [10].

In spite of their worldwide importance, the illnesses associated with heat stress and exercise have received relatively little attention in the United States. While diffuse systemic involvement has been recognized with these disorders [3], very little clinicopathological information is available concerning the renal abnormalities.

In this paper 8 cases of acute renal failure in military recruits associated with heat stress and exercise are described. Particular attention is focused on several prominent features of the clinical course, the renal histological abnormalities, and the possible etiological factors.

Methods

Lactic dehydrogenase (LDH) isoenzyme determinations [11] were kindly performed by Dr. N. M. Papadopoulos. Lactate [12] and aldolase [13] measurements were performed using the Biochemica Test combination reagent kit. The ammonium sulfate screening test was used for the detection of urine myoglobin [14]. All other determinations were performed in the hospital chemistry and hematology laboratories using standard methods.

Routine autopsy tissue sections were stained with hematoxylin eosin. In addition, the periodic acid-Schiff reaction and the benzidine reaction for hemoglobin (Pickworth) [15] were also used on all kidney sections.

Case Reports

Case 1. Patient M. J. (WRGH 7886057), a 19-year-old white male from Pittsburgh, was in good health and was active in athletics before basic training in South Carolina. He was overweight, however, and was placed on a reducing diet during the basic course. In spite of high environmental temperature and humidity, the recruit experienced no difficulties during the initial 6 weeks of training except for a skin rash over his lower extremities. However, on August 3, 1966, while on a 12-mile hike, he developed severe muscle cramps and collapsed. He was taken immediately to the dispensary and found to have a rectal temperature of 108°F, an unobtainable blood pressure, and a pulse rate of 160/min. Treatment with intravenous fluid, hydrocortisone, and metaraminol and vigorous cooling with ice packs was instituted. Although the patient's blood pressure and temperature responded to therapy, he remained confused and intermittently agitated. Initial laboratory data were hematocrit, 44 ml/100 ml; blood urea nitrogen (BUN), 75 mg/100 ml; serum sodium, 144 mEq/l; potassium, 5.8 mEq/l; and chloride, 91 mEq/l. Numerous red blood cells and white blood cells per high power field and proteinuria were found on the initial urinalysis.

During the initial 22 h after admission, the patient received 3,650 ml of fluid and 50 g of mannitol. The total urine output, however, was only 370 ml even though vasopressors were no longer needed to maintain a normal blood pressure. On the second day of hospitalization the patient's total urine output was 40 ml, and he was transferred to Walter Reed General Hospital for management of acute renal failure.

Physical examination on arrival at Walter Reed revealed proximal muscle tenderness and a scaly erythematous rash involving the anterior trunk and the legs. He remained anuric [1] during the first 14 days at Walter Reed (figure 1). Retrograde pyelograms were unremarkable. His clinical course was complicated by intermittent febrile episodes without definite clinical or cultural evidence of infection; however, chloromycetin, methicillin, and cephalothin were administered. In addition, two episodes of pulmonary edema were associated with diffuse ST-segment and T-wave changes on the electrocar-

1   Anuria shall be defined as a total 24-h urine output less than 75 ml.

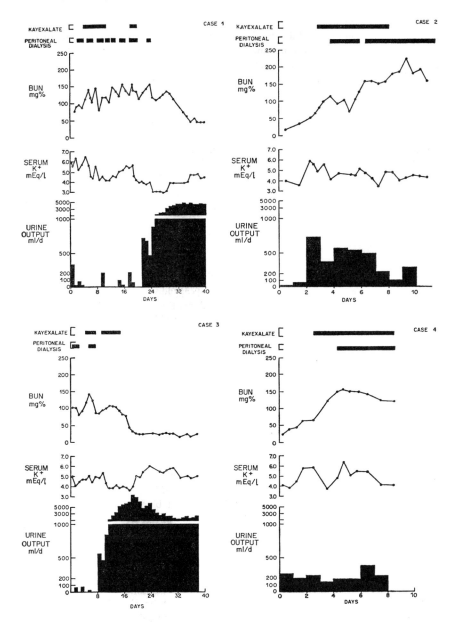

Fig. 1. Acute renal failure secondary to heat stress and exercise. BUN = blood urea nitrogen.

diogram. Concomitant hypertension required parenteral Apresoline® (hydralazine) therapy. The patient remained disoriented during the first 3 weeks of hospitalization. The neurological examination was unremarkable aside from hyperesthesia in the lower extremities. Lumbar punctures were normal except for elevated opening pressures ranging from 250 to 310 mm H_2O. Delayed nerve conduction velocity studies and the presence of denervation fibrillations on electromyographic examination suggested the presence of a peripheral neuropathy. Action potentials of very short duration (1 to 3 msec) and low amplitude (50 to 200 μV) were also demonstrated and considered evidence of a myopathy. Elevated serum glutamic-oxaloacetic transaminase (SGOT) (maximum, 557 U), aldolase [2] (maximum, 306 mU/ml), and LDH [2] (maximum, 11,500 U muscle/liver isoenzyme composed largest fraction) with normal bilirubin, alkaline phosphatase, and thymol turbidity also suggested diffuse muscle damage. Two initial urinalyses obtained at Walter Reed were negative for myoglobin and positive for hemoglobin. Plasma hemoglobin was 75 mg/ 100 ml when the initial urine was voided. Clotting studies revealed normal platelet counts and an isolated factor VII deficiency.

The patient required 8 peritoneal dialyses before a diuresis ensued on the 21st day of hospitalization. Serum creatinine returned to normal by the 33rd hospital day, and he was subsequently discharged with a normal intravenous pyelogram; BUN, 13 mg/100 ml; creatinine, 1.1 mg/100 ml; and endogenous creatinine clearance, 124 ml/min.

Case 2. Patient J. L. (WRGH 5720053), a 24-year-old white male recruit from West Virginia, had been in good health during his initial month of basic training in Kentucky. On August 28, 1960, while on a 3- to 3½-h march, he suddenly collapsed. He was taken immediately to the emergency ward in an unconscious state and was found to have a rectal temperature of 108°F and a blood pressure of 80/50 mm Hg. His clothing was saturated, and his skin was cool and moist. These observations were made, however, after attempts at cooling en route to the hospital. Vasopressors were used to sustain the patient's blood pressure, and he was packed in ice resulting in defervescence over the next 2 h. During the first few hours of hospitalization he was alternately unresponsive and agitated and, in addition, had several episodes of coffee-ground emesis and guaiac-positive liquid stools. Initial laboratory data were hematocrit, 49 ml/100 ml; hemoglobin, 17.5 g/ 100 ml; white blood cell count (WBC), 6,686/mm³; BUN, 19 mg/100 ml; serum sodium, 146 mEq/l; potassium, 4.0 mEq/l; chloride, 107 mEq/l; total carbon dioxide, 22 mEq/l.

In spite of 4 U of whole blood and 3½ l of intravenous fluids, the patient voided only 12 ml of grossly bloody urine during the first 24 h of hospitalization. Vasopressors were discontinued 6 h after admission, and subsequent blood pressures ranged from 80 to 100/50 to 70 mm Hg. On the second hospital day he was transferred to Walter Reed General Hospital. While the patient's condition was stable on departure from Kentucky, on arrival at Walter Reed he was moribund, with blood pressure of 60/0 mm Hg, pulse rate of 158/min, respirations of 48/min, and peripheral cyanosis. Many red blood cells, white blood cells, and granular casts per high power field and proteinuria were found on the initial urinalysis at Walter Reed. The hypotension improved with volume expansion and levarterenol, the latter being necessary until the 4th hospital day. Complications during the hospital course included bloody gastric drainage, disorientation, progressive jaundice (total bilirubin, 17.6 mg/ 100 ml; SGOT, 720 U), and persistent fever. Although evidence of bacterial infection was not obtained, therapy included parenteral penicillin

2   Normal values: aldolase, 0.9 to 2,5 mU/ml; LDH, 200 to 400 U.

and chloromycetin, in addition to digitalis, prochlorperazine, and hydrocortisone. Initial clotting studies included a bleeding time of 5.0 min, a clotting time of 9.0 min, and a prothrombin time of 17.4 sec (control, 12.2). Thrombocytopenia also developed later in the hospital course. Oliguria persisted, and almost constant peritoneal dialysis was necessary to control the azotemia (fig. 1).

After apparent improvement on the 8th hospital day the BUN began rising despite dialysis, and on the following day hypotension recurred. The BUN eventually reached 224 mg/100 ml although the creatinine remained stable at 6.2 mg/100 ml. This divergence between the creatinine and the BUN values was not noted in any of the other cases and was felt to be due to a gastrointestinal hemorrhage. This patent did not respond to therapy and died on the 10th hospital day.

Autopsy findings: The lungs were congested, and a single small area of pulmonary infarction was present. The left ventricle of the heart contained an area of subendocardial hemorrhage. The liver contained large regions of centrilobular necrosis. There was minimal interstitial inflammation of the head of the pancreas. Multiple gastrointestinal ulcerations that contained *Candida albicans* were found. *Candida albicans* was also cultured from the peritoneum and was considered a causal factor in the fibrinous peritonitis found at autopsy. Grossly, the musculo-skleletal system was unremarkable; however, microscopic examination of muscle was not done. Focal cerebral and cerebellar hemorrhages and cerebellar degeneration were present.

The right and left kidneys weighed 280 and 225 g, respectively. Microscopically, the glomeruli and the proximal tubules were unaltered. Distal tubules and collecting ducts in both the cortex and the medulla as well as in thin limbs of Henle's loop contained granular and homogeneous pigmented casts and occasional hyaline casts. There was a similar distribution of large calcium oxalate crystals. The latter were rarely observed in the interstitium, which was otherwise unremarkable. Many of the tubules that contained casts and crystals were atrophic. Pickworth stains revealed that many of the pigmented casts were benzidine-reactive, indicating the presence of a heme compound. The vessels were structurally unaltered although peritubular capillaries were severely congested. No evidence of frank tubular necrosis was observed.

Case 3. Patient J. B. (WRGH 7908040), a 21-year-old white male from New York City, had been physically inactive but in good health before reporting for active military duty. He arrived at an Army installation in North Carolina on August 6, 1966, and began physical training 2 days later during high environmental temperatures. The recruit tolerated the training until August 20 when he became weak, confused, and febrile to 104°F after strenuous physical exercise. After being hospitalized for 2 days with the diagnosis of 'viral syndrome,' he was discharged. Two days later the recruit noted severe muscle cramps and collapsed during a 1½- to 2-mile march. On admission to the hospital he was described as warm and exhausted with a rectal temperauure of 103.2°F. The blood pressure was initially 110/70 mm Hg, on arrival at the medical ward the pressure had decreased to 90/70 mm Hg. Initial laboratory data were hematocrit, 55 ml/100 ml; hemoglobin, 18.2 g/100 ml; WBC, 20, 207/mm³; BUN, less than 10 mg/100 ml; SGOT, 900 U; and normal bilirubin and alkaline phosphatase. The urine was positive with Hematest® stick and contained protein, 6 to 8 red blood cells/hpf, hemoglobin casts, and white blood cell casts.

The patient remained anuric in spite of fluid replacement, and on the 3rd hospital day he was transferred to Walter Reed General Hospital with a BUN of 90 mg/100 ml;

serum sodium, 124 mEq/l; potassium, 5.0 mEq/l; chloride, 80 mEq/l; and total carbon dioxide, 25 mEq/l. On arrival at Walter Reed he complained of mild myalgia. The only abnormal physical finding was a blood pressure of 160/100 mm Hg. His subsequent course included 7 further days of anuria (fig. 1). Retrograde pyleograms did not reveal obstruction. SGOT and LDH determinations revealed maximal values of 1,016 and 1,025 U, respectively, with normal cephalin flocculation, thymol turbidity, bilirubin, and alkaline phosphatase. Platelet counts, prothrombin time, and partial thromboplastin time were normal.

After 11 days and two 36-h peritoneal dialyses the patient entered the diuretic phase. Serum creatinine had returned to normal by the 66th hospital day, and he was subsequently discharged with a serum creatinine of 1.4 mg/100 ml and an endogenous creatinine clearance of 157 ml/min.

Case 4. Patient G. S. (WRGH 7176064),[3] a 22-year-old white male from northern Wisconsin, reported to Georgia for basic training on August 19, 1964. The recruit had been in good health except for a 25-lb weight gain over the previous 2 years. During the first 2 days of his basic training environmental temperature and humidity were quite high, and no physical exercises were conducted. However, on August 21 the temperature was only 77°F, and he participated in a 1- to 1½-mile march. After returning to his barracks, he became confused and agitated. He was taken immediately to the emergency room and was noted to have hot, dry skin and a rectal temperature of 108°F. The patient was placed in an ice bath and given intravenous chlorpromazine. A grand mal seizure accompanied by hypotension occurred shortly after the initiation of this therapy.

On transfer to the ward his blood pressure was 90/70 mm Hg, and initial laboratory data were hematocrit, 50 ml/100 ml; hemoglobin, 16.1 g/100 ml; BUN, 22.5 mg/100 ml; WBC, 9,342/mm³; serum sodium, 148 mEq/l; potassium, 4.1 mEq/l; chloride, 115 mEq/l; and total carbon dioxide, 23 mEq/l. Urinalysis showed proteinuria, many red blood cells, and coarse granular casts. The supernatant was negative for myoglobin and hemoglobin with benzidine reagent.

During the first 24 h of hospitalization the urine output was only 225 ml in spite of a total fluid intake of 3,600 ml and 3 trials with 12.5 g mannitol intravenously. His temperature was controlled with a cooling mattress, and blood pressure was maintained with intravenous metaraminol during his initial 3 days of hospitalization. On the 3rd hospital day intramuscular penicillin was begun due to the suspicion of pneumonia. Persistent oliguria, an obtundent mental status, and the development of jaundice in conjunction with a BUN of 66 mg/100 ml, serum potassium of 5.9 mEq/l, and total carbon dioxide of 9 mEq/l prompted transfer to Walter Reed General Hospital on the 4th hospital day.

On arrival at Walter Reed the patient's blood pressure was 96/60 mm Hg, and his rectal temperature was 100.4°F. Acneiform lesions were present on the trunk and the lower extremities, and blisters were noted on the volar surface of the hands and the feet. The lungs were clear to auscultation, and a chest film was unremarkable. Continuous peritoneal dialysis was instituted on the 2nd hospital day and maintained the BUN below 150 mg/100 ml (fig. 1). His temperature remained labile, requiring a cooling mattress, and intravenous metaraminol was needed intermittently to maintain normal

---

3   This case report was published in 'Military Medicine', August 1966, by Dr. Jack W. COBURN and is included in the present study with the permission of the author and the journal.

blood pressures. Liver function tests were markedly abnormal: total bilirubin, 19.5mg/ 100 ml; alkaline phosphatase, 17.6 King-Armstrong U; SGOT, 1,070 U; and cephalin flocculation, 4+. In addition, a diminished platelet count of 80,000 was accompanied by a prolonged prothrombin time; however, no clinical evidence of bleeding occurred. Although the patient's level of consciousness had improved and the degree of jaundice had lessened, on the 9th hospital day he apparently aspirated and could not be resuscitated.

Autopsy findings: The lungs showed pulmonary congestion and edema with an early bronchopneumonia in both lower lobes. A focal area of subendocardial hemorrhage was found in the right ventricle of the heart. Diffuse central and midzonal degeneration of hepatic parenchymal cells was present. The cerebral cortex and the basal ganglion showed marked hyperemia without neuronal degeneration. Focal vacuolization and degeneration of skeletal muscle were present.

The right and left kidneys weighed 380 and 340 g, respectively. Microscopically, the glomeruli, the larger vessels, and the interstitium were unremarkable. In both cortical and medullary regions numerous pigmented granular casts were observed in distal tubules and collecting ducts. Similar casts were present in many atrophic unidentifiable tubules in the cortex and in thin loops of Henle in the medulla. Because of *post-mortem* alterations, unequivocal areas of tubular necrosis were not identifiable. Many peritubular capillaries contained collections of mononuclear cells and were severely congested.

Case 5. Patient R. G. (WRGH 6791078), a 23-year-old white male from northern Virginia, began basic training on July 24, 1963, in Georgia. Before induction he was in good health but had been employed in a sedentary job in an air-conditioned building. During the 1st day of basic training the temperature and the humidity were quite high, and the recruit complained of profuse sweating, weakness, and dizziness. He reported to the outpatient clinic and was encouraged to increase his salt and fluid intake.

One week later returned with similar complaints and related taking salt tablets but little water. He was confused, anhidrotic, and severely dehydrated, with a blood pressure of 80/60 mm Hg, a pulse rate of 120/min, and a temperature of 99°F. Initial laboratory data were hematocrit, 48 ml/100 ml; hemoglobin, 16.0 g/100 ml; WBC, 9,400/mm^3; BUN, 55 mg/100 ml; creatinine, 3.7 mg/100 ml; serum sodium, 168 mEq/l; potassium, 5.3 mEq/l; chloride, 143 mEq/l; and total carbon dioxide, 28.0 mEq/l.[4] Proteinuria, 7 to 9 red blood cells and 10 to 12 white blood cells/hpf, and granular casts were noted on initial urinalysis.

Although no therapy had been instituted on arrival at the medical ward, blood pressure had increased to 130/80 mm Hg. Total urine output during the first 56 h of hospitalization was only 590 ml in spite of the administration of almost 10 l of dextrose in water. The patient's temperature rose to 103°F rectally without evidence of infection. Oliguria persisted, and by the 5th hospital day the BUN had risen to 140 mg/100 ml, prompting transfer to Walter Reed General Hospital.

On arrival at Walter Reed his temperature was 99.6°F and his blood pressure, 128/ 72 mm Hg. The patient was confused without focal neurologic signs and had a maculo-papular rash over the chest and back. Peritoneal dialysis was instituted, and 100 exchanges were carried out over the next 5 days (fig. 2). BUN decreased from 202 to 71 mg/100 ml; however, the patient remained confused and disoriented. The following day he became

---

4   Repeated determinations confirmed electrolyte abnormalities: sodium, 160 mEq/l; potassium, 5.5 mEq/l; chloride, 132 mEq/l; total carbon dioxide, 26 mEq/l.

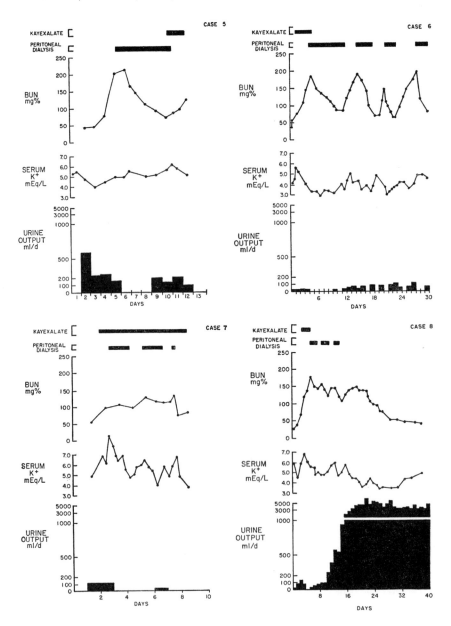

Fig. 2. Acute renal failure secondary to heat stress and exercise. BUN = blood urea nitrogen.

febrile and developed respiratory difficulty. Penicillin, streptomycin, oxytetracycline, and, later, methicillin were administered for a suspected pneumonia. A tracheostomy was performed with improvement in respirations, but the patient's temperature rose to 103°F. His blood pressure also increased to 180/120 mm Hg, and bilateral papilledema and retinal hemorrhages appeared. The following day the patient died in acute pulmonary edema that did not respond to the use of tourniquets, phlebotomy, and peritoneal dialysis with hypertonic glucose.

Clotting studies during his course revealed a normal prothrombin time and a platelet count of 80,000/mm³. Liver function studies became abnormal preterminally: total bilirubin, 1.2 mg/100 ml; SGOT, 64 U; alkaline phosphatase, 85.0 King-Armstrong U; total protein, 5.3 g/100 ml; and albumin, 2.6 g/100 ml.

Autopsy findings: The thorax contained 2.5 l of fluid and the abdomen, 1.0 l. The lungs weighed over, 2,000 g and contained large amounts of frothy edema. The liver was moderately congested and had focal areas of centrilobular necrosis. The cerebral cortex was moderately congested and edematous and showed focal neuronal degeneration. There was a 20% loss of Purkinje's cells in the cerebellum. No microscopic examination of skeletal muscle was undertaken.

The right and left kidneys weighed 190 and 200 g, repectively. The glomeruli, the larger vessels, and the proximal tubules were unremarkable. Occasional granular pigmented casts were scattered throughout the kidney in the distal tubules, the collecting ducts, and the thin loops of Henle. Many of these casts reacted in a positive manner with the Pickworth stain. There was no evidence of tubular necrosis or regeneration. Many peritubular capillaries within the medulla contained foci of mononucleated white blood cells and were generally congested.

Case 6. Patient J. B. (WRGH 6789053), a 23-year-old white male from Illinois, had been unemployed and inactive for 2 years before his induction into the military service. On July 22, 1963, he reported for basic training in Kentucky, and vigorous physical exercise began on July 31 during an environmental temperature in excess of 90°F. The following evening the recruit felt weak, hot, and dizzy and complained of a severe, generalized, throbbing headache. The next morning he passed a small quantity of reddish-brown urine, and in the early afternoon he suddenly became confused and collapsed.

Immediately after being sponged with cool water the patient was taken to the hospital in a semicomatose and combative condition. His skin was hot and dry, his blood pressure was 140/80 mm Hg, and his temperature was 102.8°F. However, within 45 min it had risen to 105.8°F. Initial laboratory data were hemoglobin, 15.8 g/100 ml; hematocrit, 48ml/100 ml; WBC, 16,750/mm³; BUN, 40 mg/100 ml; sodium, 150 mEq/l; potassium, 4.7 mEq/l; chloride, 120 mEq/l; and total carbon dioxide, 17.5 mEq/l. Urinalysis revealed innumerable red blood cells and white blood cells per high power field, granular casts, and protein.

In spite of the intravenous administration of 4,000 ml of 5% dextrose in water, 1,000 ml of 5% dextrose in isotonic saline, and 12.5 g of mannitol during the first 18 h, the total urine output was only 40 ml. On arrival at Walter Reed General Hospital the following day he was alert, with a blood pressure of 130/90 mm Hg and a papulopustular rash on the neck and the trunk. On the 2nd hospital day, however, the blood pressure fell to 85/50 mm Hg, and vasopressors and penicillin, chloromycetin, and streptomycin therapy were initiated because of possible gram-negative bacteremia. Vasopressors were discontinued the following day, but the antibiotics were continued for 21 days. His course was characterized by 30 days of anuria requiring frequent peritoneal dialysis (fig. 2). A persistent low-grade fever with positive peritoneal cultures for *Klebsiella-Aerobacter* was found. An episode of marked hypertension (blood pressure, 170/120 mm Hg) with papilledema and retinal hemorrhages occurred on the 14th hospital day, and gastrointestinal bleeding manifested by guaic-positive stools complicated the final 2 weeks of the hospital course. Liver function studies were essentially normal throughout the entire illness. Clotting studies (prothrombin time and platelet count) were initially normal, but thrombocytopenia developed on the 16th hospital day. On the 24th hospital day the patient's temperature rose to 103°F, and the blood cultures grew *Candida albicans.* Three days later hypothermia was initiated as potential therapy for the yeast septicemia; however, the patient developed hypotension and died on the 30th hospital day.

Autopsy findings: The lungs revealed mild pulmonary edema. The pancreas was diffusely involved with a suppurative inflammatory process. Gastric and colonic ulcers were present, and there was centrilobular necrosis of the liver. There was a diffuse fibro-purulent peritonitis. Microabscesses were present in kidneys, brain, heart, and muscles. In addition, there was extensive rhabdomyolysis with marked calcification involving predominantly the proximal skeletal musculature and, to a lesser extent, the distal musculature.

The right and left kidneys weighed 210 and 200 g, respectively. Their surface was covered with microabscesses. Microscopically, the abscesses represented foci of tubules and adjacent glomeruli involved in an acute suppurative inflammatory process. The glomeruli, the vessels, and the interstitium were otherwise unaltered. Numerous distal tubules and collecting ducts throughout the kidneys contained pigmented granular and occasional hyaline casts. Many of the casts stained positive with the Pickworth stain. Intratubular crystals of calcium oxalate were also observed. Except in the regions of microabscess formation, evidence of frank tubular necrosis was not present. Peritubular capillaries within the medulla were congested. *Candida* was cultured from the blood and observed microscopically in the renal microabscesses.

Case 7. Patient P. T. (WRGH 7895030), a 19-year-old white male from New York, was overweight but otherwise in good health until 2nd week of basic training at a military installation in North Carolina. On August 11, 1966, after participating in physical training exercises, he became irrational and collapsed in the barracks. On arriving at the hospital the patient had hot, dry skin, was disoriented with slurred speech, and complained of leg pain. His temperature was 103.8°F, respirations, 20/min, and blood pressure, 130/90 mm Hg. Initial laboratory data were hematocrit, 48 ml/100 ml; hemoglobin, 17.7 g/100 ml; WBC, 11,094/mm³; BUN, 59 mg/100 ml; sodium, 143 mEq/l; potassium, 4.9 mEq/l; chloride, 116 mEq/l; and total carbon dioxide, 19.5 mEq/l. The initial urine was dark brown and positive for protein. Microscopic examination revealed many coarsely granular and red blood cell casts and numerous red blood cells per high power field.

The patient remained markedly oliguric in spite of therapy with intravenous fluids, corticosteroids, and mannitol. On the 3rd hospital day the BUN had risen to over 100 mg/100 ml, and the potassium was 6.9 mEq/l. The patient was transferred to Walter Reed General Hospital.

On arrival at Walter Reed he was obtunded, his skin was cold and clammy, his rectal temperature was 106°F, and his blood pressure was 160/120 mm Hg. The temperature shortly rose to 107°F, and treatment with a cooling mattress resulted in reduction to normal levels over the next 1½ h. However, a low-grade fever persisted during his entire hospital course. Although cultural evidence of infection could not be obtained, parenteral cephalothin and, later, chloromycetin were administered. The patient remained anuric, and 2 peritoneal dialyses were performed (fig. 2), the 2nd complicated by an intra-abdominal hemorrhage. Subsequently, a 6-h hemodialysis was more effective in correcting the biochemical abnormalities. Nevertheless, the patient's mental status progressively worsened. Localizing neurologic signs were absent, and 2 examinations of the cerebrospinal fluid were normal. Sustained hypertension persisted and was treated with parenteral reserpine. Clotting studies including prothrombin time, partial thromboplastin time, fibrinogen level, and platelet counts were within normal limits. Diffuse muscle damage was suggested by extremely high serum enzyme elevations including SGOT (maximum, 2,250 U), aldolase (maximum, 500 Um/ml), and LDH (maximum, 22,000 U—muscle/ liver isoenzyme composed largest fraction), with normal bilirubin and alkaline phosphatase.

On the 8th hospital day respiratory difficulties appeared, and despite tracheostomy and assisted ventilation the patient had a cardiac arrest and died on the 9th hospital day.

Autopsy findings: Examination of the lungs revealed diffuse moderate edema and a mucopurulent bronchitis. An acute fibropurulent bronchopneumonia was present in the right middle lobe. The heart and the liver were unremarkable. Moderate cerebral edema was found, with slight diffuse neuronal degeneration. Extensive rhabdomyolysis was present, especially in proximal muscle groups (fig. 3).

The right and left kidneys weighed 280 and 260 g, respectively. The glomeruli and the vessels were unremarkable (fig. 4). Many granular pigmented casts were present in distal tubules and collecting ducts in both the cortex and the medulla and in thin loops of Henle in the medulla (fig. 5). The majority of the casts reacted positively when sections were stained according to the method of Pickworth. There was no evidence of tubular necrosis. Mild to moderate edema of the medullary area was present, and marked congestion of peritubular capillaries was observed. Otherwise the interstitium was unremarkable.

Case 8. Patient A. P. (WRGH 7881039), a 21-year-old Negro male from New York City, had been in good health but physically inactive before beginning his active reserve status in New Jersey. He started physical exercise on July 11, 1966, and had difficulty in completing running exercise. Otherwise he felt well until July 25 when, while finishing a 2-mile run, he suddenly became weak, dizzy, and collapsed. He was taken immediately to the emergency room where he regained consciousness and complained of severe thirst and muscle cramps. His skin was cold and clammy, and his blood pressure was 100/60 mm Hg with a pulse rate of 130/min. After 2 l of isotonic saline intravenously and a quart of orange juice orally, he was discharged to his barracks. However, the patient collapsed again en route to his barracks and was admitted to the hospital. He was noted to be anhidrotic with a temperature of 101°F and hypotensive with a systolic pressure of 60 to 70 mm Hg. During the first 24 h of hospitalization, he had multiple episodes of profuse, guaiac-positive watery diarrhea associated with generalized abdominal and muscle pain. His blood pressure rose to normal, but in spite of 5,000 ml of fluid and 37.5 g of mannitol intravenously he remained anuric, with a total output of 20 ml 'bloody' urine during the first 24 h of hospitalization.

Initial laboratory data were hematocrit, 58 ml/100 ml; WBC, 24,000/mm³; BUN, 24 mg/100 ml; sodium, 135 mEq/l; chloride, 103 mEq/l; potassium, 4.3 mEq/l; and total carbon dioxide, 16 mEq/l. Innumerable red blood cells per high power field, granular casts, and protein were found on initial urinalysis. Retrograde pyelograms were performed and no obstruction was observed. On July 27 the patient's total bilirubin was 2.3 mg/

Table I Clinical features of nephropathy associated with heat stress and exercise [a]

Case No.	Age, race, sex (yr)	Duration of prior physical training (days)	Rectal temperature (F)	Blood pressure (mm Hg)	Hematocrit Hemoglobin % g/100 ml	Neurological manifestations
1	19, white, M	42	108	Unobtainable	44	Confusion, agitation, peripheral neuropathy
2	24, white, M	28	108	80/50	49 17.5	Coma, then confusion and agitation
3	21, white, M	14	103.2	110/70 [d]	55 18.2	Confusion
4	22, white, M	2	108	90/70	50 16.1	Convulsion, confusion
5	23, white, M	7	99	80/60	48 16.0	Confusion
6	23, white, M	1	102.8 [e]	140/80	48 15.8	Semicomatose, agitation
7	19, white, M	10	103,8	130/90	48 17.7	Coma, then confusion
8	21, Negro, M	14	101	60/0	58	Coma, then confusion

[a] *Post-mortem* findings in fatal cases presented in case reports.
[b] EMG = electromyogram; SGOT = serum glutamic-oxaloacetic transaminase; LDH = lactic dehydrogenase.
[c] Catheterized specimen.

Clinical evidence of muscle damage [b]	Extrarenal manifestations	Urine abnormalities	Outcome
Muscle cramps, abnormal EMG, elevated aldolase, SGOT, and LDH	Acute pulmonary edema, electro-cardiogramm and clotting abnormalities hemoglobinemia, skin rash, hypertension, persistent fever	Proteinuria,[c] hematuria, pyuria, hemoglobin–positive, myoglobin–negative	Recovered
None	Hepatic necrosis with marked jaundice, thrombocytopenia, clotting abnormalities, persistent fever, gastrointestinal hemorrhage	Proteinuria,[c] hematuria, pyuria, cylindruria	Died on 10th hospital day in shock
Muscle cramps, elevated SGOT and LDH	Hypertension	Proteinuria,[c] hematuria, hemo-globin and white blood cell casts	Recovered
None	Hepatic necrosis with severe jaundice, thrombocytopenia, clotting abnormalities, skin rash, persistent fever	Proteinuria,[c] hematuria, granular casts, hemoglobin–negative, myoglobin–negative	Died on 9th hospital day of respiratory complication
None	Skin rash, persistent fever, hypertension with papilledema, pulmonary edema	Proteinuria,[c] hematuria, pyuria, granular casts	Died on 11th hospital day in pulmonary edema
None	Skin rash, hypertension with papilledema, persistent fever, thrombocytopenia, gastrointestinal hemorrhage	Proteinuria,[c] hematuria, pyuria, granular casts	Died on 13th hospital day with candida septicemia
Muscle cramps, elevated aldolase, SGOT, and LDH	Hypertension, persistent fever	Proteinuria,[c] hematuria, granular and red blood cell casts	Died on 9th hospital day of respiratory and cardiac arrest
Muscle cramps	Diarrhea, hepatic necrosis with severe jaundice	Proteinuria,[c] hematuria, granular casts	Recovered

[d]   Blood pressure had decreased to 90/70 mm Hg when patient arrived on medical ward.
[e]   Initial temperature taken after sponging with cool water; increased to 105.8°F within 45 min.

100 ml, and SGOT was greater than 2,000 U. A liver biopsy demonstrated parenchyma necrosis and acute inflammation predominantly in a peripheral zonal location. The patient remained anuric with an increase in BUN to 130 mg/100 ml and serum potassium to 6.0 mg/100 ml, and on July 30 he was transferred to Walter Reed General Hospital for management of acute renal failure. The anuria persisted for a total of 10 days (fig. 2), and oliguria was present for 5 more days, necessitating peritoneal dialysis on three occasions until a diuresis ensued. Coagulation studies including prothrombin time, platelet count, and partial thromboplastin time were within normal limits. A sickle cell preparation was positive, and hemoglobin SA was demonstrated by electrophoresis. Hepatic function returned to normal. The BUN returned to 21 mg/100 ml by the 59th hospital day, and he was subsequently discharged with a BUN of 21 mg/100 ml, a creatinine of 1.5 mg/100 ml, and a creatinine clearance of 133 ml/min. An intravenous pyelogram exhibited a bifid left ureter as the only abnormality.

Summary of Clinical Features

Eight patients with acute renal failure associated with heat stress and physical exertion were treated at Walter Reed General Hospital between 1960 and 1966 (table 1). The predisposing factors and the onset of illness were very similar in every instance. Every case occurred during the summer months, and most of the recruits had lived in the northern United States and were undergoing basic training in the southern United States. The majority were overweight and had been physically inactive before induction into the Army. In 6 of the 8 cases the onset of illness occurred during the first 2 weeks of basic training. The age of the patients ranged from 19 to 24 years, and 7 of the 8 were white. The only Negro (Case 8) was atypical in that he underwent training in northern United States, had sickle cell trait, and possibly had antecedent viral hepatitis. Before their present illness, all of the patients had had one or more normal induction urine examinations and blood pressure recordings, and none had a history of cardiac or renal disease. Atropine-like medications that would interfere with heat-regulating mechanisms had not been ingested, and recent immunizations could not be incriminated. There was also no previous history of episodes of muscle cramps and dark urine. Lactate production studies were performed during ischemic and non-ischemic forearm exercise in 3 patients (table II). These studies were undertaken during the convalescent period after recovery from acute renal failure. All 3 patients increased their lactate blood levels during exercise, thus excluding a phosphorylase deficiency such as McArdle's syndrome [16].

The onset of the illness was either abrupt or was preceded by 1 to 7 days of premonitory symptoms such as weakness, dizziness, or muscle cramps. Sudden collapse, convulsions, agitation, or disorientation were consistent features of the acute illness, and initial hypotension was found in 6 patients. The patients' skin was generally described as hot and dry, and rectal temperature elevations of 103.2°F or greater were found during the first hour of hospitalization in all but 2 of the patients. Skin rashes were present in 4 cases.

Admission laboratory data revealed evidence of hemoconcentration in 7 cases (hematocrit, 48 to 58%; hemoglobin, 15.8 to 18.2 g/100 ml) and leukocytosis in 4. The initial blood urea nitrogen (BUN) was elevated in 6 cases (23 to 75 mg/100 ml). Three patients presented with the total carbon dioxide values below 20 mEq/l, but none of the patients had initial hypo- or hyperkalemia. Severe hypernatremia occurred in 1 case.

The subsequent hospital course and the *post-mortem* examination in the 5 fatal cases provided evidence for the generalized nature of the illness. Persistent abnormalities of cerebral function without focal neurologic signs were a prominent feature in 5 patients. Lumbar punctures were unremarkable except for elevated opening pressures in several instances. Cerebral congestion and focal hemorrhages were found at *post-mortem* examination in 4 patients. Cardiac abnormalities were detected clinically in 1 patient and on *post-mortem* examination in 2 other patients. Four patients had clinical evidence of liver damage or centrilobular necrosis on *post-mortem* examination or both. Severe hypotension and prolonged use of vasopressors had occurred in 3 of these cases. Evidence of pancreatitis was found at autopsy in 2 patients. Gastrointestinal hemorrhage occurred in 3 cases. Gastrointestinal ulcerations were found at autopsy in 2 of these patients, and the cause of the hemorrhage was not established in the other surviving patient. Coagulation abnormalities or thrombocytopenia was noted in 5 patients.

Table II. Lactate production during ischemic and nonischemic forearm exercise.

	Case 1	Case 3	Case 8
		(mg/100 ml)	
Control	12.1	14.2	15.6
5-min nonischemic exercise	35.9	50.3	67.2
1-h postexercise.	7.4	10.8	14.8
1-min ischemic exercise	15.9	31.0	33.6

Four patients developed marked hypertension, and 2 of these patients also had papilledema. Fever persisted throughout the hospital course in 5 patients without clear-cut evidence of bacterial infection.

A prominent feature of the illness, also recently observed by others [17], was the muscle damage (fig. 3). A history of severe muscle cramps was obtained from 4 patients. In 3 patients marked elevation of serum enzymes including aldolase, serum glutamic-oxaloacetic transaminase (SGOT), and lactic dehydrogenase (LDH) occurred concomitantly with normal liver function studies. In 2 of the latter cases the LDH isoenzyme most markedly elevated was the skeletal muscle/liver group, end, in addition, one of these patients had electromyographic evidence of myopathy. Histologic evidence of diffuse muscle damage including vacuolization, degeneration, and extensive rhabdomyolysis was found in 3 of the fatal cases.

The illness frequently presented with the excretion of small amounts of reddish-brown urine, and initial urinalyses usually revealed proteinuria, cylindruria, hematuria, and pyuria. On 2 occasions screening tests were negative for myoglobin. Anuria (24-h urine volumes less than 75 ml) was a prominent feature in 5 cases for periods ranging from 8 to 32 days. These

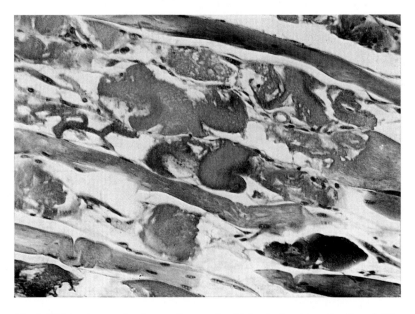

Fig. 3. Light micrograph of necrotic muscle obtained at autopsy in *Case 7*. The tissue was removed from the quadriceps muscle. Hematoxylin-eosin stain, × 180.

periods of anuria were unassociated with hypotension, volume depletion, or use of vasopressors, and retrograde pyelograms or *post-mortem* examination excluded significant obstruction. In some of the patients there was apparent hypercatabolism, reflected by the need for cation-exchange resins and frequent dialysis to control the hyperkalemia and thea zotemia. Only 3 patients entered the diuretic phase, and each one of them survived. The ultimate renal function in each instance appeared to be normal as measured by endogenous creatinine clearance.

Of the 5 patients that died, 2 died with respiratory problems after prolonged coma, 1 with hypotension (probably secondary to gastrointestinal bleeding), 1 with pulmonary edema, and 1 with candida sepsis.

Discussion

The clinical spectrum and classification of heat disorders were well summarized recently by LEITHEAD and LIND [18]. By definition, hyperpyrexia is necessary to classify a case as 'classical heatstroke,' and the acceptable lower limit of temperature elevation has varied from 103 to 106°F [4–7]. In the present series 2 unacclimatized recruits developed acute renal failure after strenuous exercise in a hot environment, although they did not present with documented temperature elevations in excess of 103°F. They have been included, however, since the circumstances and the clinical course of their illness were otherwise indistinguishable from those of the other patients' illnesses. The best classification for the entire group is probably 'renal failure secondary to heat stress and exercise.'

Clinical renal abnormalities have been mentioned in a number of large series [3–7, 9] of heat disorders. However, these abnormalities have been of a nonspecific nature including mild azotemia, proteinuria, pyuria, hematuria, and cylindruria. Very few well-documented cases of clinical acute renal failure with heat disorders can be found in the literature. In 1949, MARCHARD and REIMER [19] reported the first documented case in a patient with luetic disease receiving fever therapy. Ten days of marked oliguria and rising azotemia were followed by a diuretic period and return of normal renal function. BAXTER and TESCHAN [20] reported 3 cases of 'atypical heatstroke' with fulminating hyperkalemia; however, they noted that only 1 patient had oliguria after blood volume had been reconstituted and vasopressor therapy had become unncessary. In the patient reported by KNOCHEL *et al.* [21] oliguria and azotemia persisted for more than 40 days, and

8 hemodialyses were performed before the patient died from a massive gastrointestinal hemorrhage. BARRY and KING [9] cited a 'few cases' of oliguric renal failure in the South African gold mines, and KEW *et al.*[22] reported 3 additional cases. VERTEL and KNOCHEL [17] have collected 10 cases of acute renal failure with heat injury at Brooke Army Medical Center during the past 8 years.

Although less than 20 documented cases of acute renal failure after heat stress and exercise have been reported in the literature, the actual incidence may be higher. Eight cases were seen at Walter Reed General Hospital between 1960 and 1966, and 4 of these patients were admitted during the past summer. The larger number of recruits involved in basic military training no doubt accounts for this apparent increased incidence. Since this increased incidence may persist, emphasis of several clinical features characteristic of this type of renal failure may be useful.

Clinical Course of Acute Renal Failure

As seen in figures 1 and 2, hyperkalemia was often a problem early in the hospital course, requiring both cation-exchange resins and frequent dialysis. The daily increment in BUN from the day of admission to the day of the first dialysis was 30 mg/100 ml or greater in 6 cases. In addition, the BUN was often difficult to control, requiring frequent and, in some cases, continuous peritoneal dialysis. These findings suggested significant hyper-catabolism[5] similar to that seen in posttraumatic renal insufficiency [23]. The multiple system involvement including the high incidence of muscle damage probably contributed to this hypercatabolic state.

The widespread organ system involvement further complicated the management of these patients. The depression of the central nervous system was disproportionately severe for the degree of azotemia and generally indicated a poorer prognosis. This obtundent mental status made supportive care, particularly the respiratory management, more difficult. Respiratory complications were actually the immediate cause of death in 2 of the fatal cases. While prophylactic antibiotics have been recommended in cases of heatstroke with prolonged coma [24], the present study would not support this therapeutic approach. The frequency of persistent temperature eleva-

5   Frequent peritoneal dialysis is indicative of hypercatabolism only if peritoneal clearance is normal. Peritoneal urea clearances were measured in Patient 6 during the 2nd week of hospitalization and were normal (14–24 ml/min).

tions complicated the clinical evaluation of infection; and, although bacterial cultures were usually negative, the fear of occult infections prompted the use of broad-spectrum antibiotics in several instances. The course of the fever was generally unaltered by the administration of these antibiotics. Furthermore, the occurrence of systemic candidiasis in 2 of the fatal cases suggested that the judicious use of antibiotics is necessary. Adequate tracheal drainage and ventilation would seem to be the most important aspects of the respiratory management.

In 4 of the patients the initial hypotension was not a problem after the lowering of body temperature, but in 3 patients hypotension required prolonged use of vasopressors. The cause of this persistent hypotension was unclear; however, myocardial damage, actual volume depletion, and peripheral vasodilatation with relative volume depletion may have all been etiological factors. Volume expanders as well as vasopressors may therefore be necessary in these patients. However, since myocardial damage also occurs, careful monitoring of this fluid replacement is necessary. Episodes of acute pulmonary edema were noted in 2 cases. In one of these patients the onset of the pulmonary edema occurred during volume replacement and was the immediate cause of death.

The presence of hypertension in 5 of the patients may not have been a greater incidence than found in acute renal failure of other etiologies [23, 25]. However, the concomitant cardiac complications made these blood pressure elevations potentially more dangerous. The 2 patients who had episodes of acute pulmonary edema also had significant hypertension. The associated papilledema in 2 cases may have been predominantly due to the hypertension, but the frequency of cerebral edema in these patients may predispose to this complication.

Other complications that had less clinical significance in these patients were liver damage, pancreatitis, and clotting abnormalities. Hepatic functional derangement with marked jaundice occurred in only 2 cases. No spontaneous hemorrhagic complications were related to the clotting abnormalities, but diffuse petechiae were noted on *post-mortem* examination in some of the fatal cases. The 2 serious instances of hemorrhage were associated with gastro-intestinal ulcers, and the other patient with gastrointestinal hemorrhage had normal clotting studies.

Another interesting characteristic of the acute renal failure was the high incidence and the long duration of urine volumes less than 75 ml/day (fig. 1 and 2). The mean daily urine output in 23 patients with acute renal failure reported by LOUGHRIDGE, MILNE, SHACKMAN, and WOOTON [26] was 75 ml during the first 6 days of oliguria and 150 ml during the entire oliguric period (24-h urine volume less than 400 ml). In the present series daily urine volumes less than 75 ml occurred in 5 cases and persisted from 7 to 32 days. Such severe and prolonged oliguria, which has been arbitrarily defined as anuria, may suggest acute necrotizing glomerulonephritis, acute renal vascular catastrophes, or excretory obstructive disease as potential causes of the acute renal failure. Since the latter 2 entities may be remediable by surgical procedures, further diagnostic studies including renal biopsy, aortography, and retrograde pyelography may be indicated. However, when marked oliguria is associated with the renal failure secondary to heat stress and exercise, it would seem advisable to be more conservative in pursuing these potentially dangerous diagnostic procedures. The severe oliguria in the present patients may be in some way related to primary renal lesion, but another alternative explanation would be the use of frequent dialysis.

The 3 patients who survived the acute renal failure had return of normal renal function as measured by endogenous creatinine clearances. This finding is in agreement with the observations of VERTEL and KNOCHEL [17]

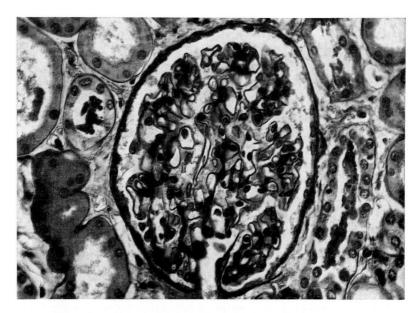

Fig. 4. Light micrograph of kidney tissue obtained at autopsy in *Case 7.* The glomerulus and the proximal convoluted tubules are unremarkable. Note the pigmented casts in an adjacent collecting duct to the left of the glomerulus and in a probable distal tubule to the right of the glomerulus. Periodic acid-Schiff stain, × 925.

in which the 7 patients who survived had return of normal renal function. In contradistinction to this finding in the American military are the findings of KEW et al. [22] in South African gold miners. They described progressive abnormalities on renal biopsy and persistent functional defects in some of their patients who suffered heatstroke. It is not clear, however, if the 2 patients who actually survived acute oliguric renal failure had persistent functional defects.

Renal Pathological Findings

The renal pathology from the 5 fatal cases reviewed by one of us (C. C. T.). The pathologic findings were similar in all 5 instances, and alterations were not extensive. Grossly, the kidneys appeared swollen and were considerably larger than normal. Microscopically, there were no significant vascular or glomerular alterations. These findings differed from a previous study by SOBEL et al. [27] of 14 patients with heatstroke. These authors reported numerous glomerular alterations including focal glomerular capillary basement membrane thickening, adhesions of the glomerular tuft to Bowman's capsule, glomerular hypercellularity, and occasional crescent formation. No evidence of clinical acute renal failure in these patients was cited. In the similar study of 17 South African gold miners with heatstroke [22] the authors also reported glomerular basement membrane thickening and prominence of epithelial cells. The differences in the glomerular findings of these 2 earlier studies when compared to our own study may be explained in part by the difference in interpretation of certain glomerular findings. Recent studies [28, 29] of nondiseased human glomeruli suggested that glomerular basement membrane thickening of a focal nature is commonly present. Thus, the significance of this finding in various disease states is not clear. The possibility that the renal effects of heat stress were superimposed on preexisting renal disease is still another explanation for the difference in findings from those of the present study. Glomerular lesions specifically related to heat stress and exercise might be anticipated to be most marked in patients with severe clinical renal disease. The lesions reported by KEW et al. [22] and by SOBEL et al. [27] were seen in a group of 31 patients with heatstroke, only 3 of whom had oliguric renal failure. In contrast, the renal pathological findings in the present series were derived from the 5 fatal cases with severe oliguric renal failure, and yet no significant glomerular abnormalities were found. In addition, these findings are in agreement with those of MALAMUD *et al.* [3], VERTEL and KNOCHEL [17], BAXTER and TESCHAN [20], and KNOCHEL *et al.* [21] who also observed the absence of glomerular lesions in fatal heatstroke.

Our material also demonstrates the lack of correlation between acute anuric or oliguric renal failure and histological tubular necrosis. Evidence of widespread tubular necrosis was not observed, regardless of the interval between the onset of the acute illness or of subsequent hypotensive episodes and the time of death. Classically, clinicians have equated acute renal parenchymal failure with tubular necrosis. LUCKE [30] first described the picture of 'lower nephron nephrosis' in 1946 after observing tubular necrosis of the distal nephron in cases of renal failure secondary to traumatic shock, burns, transfusions, blackwater fever, heatstroke, and other entities. Later, OLIVER, MACDOWELL, and TRACEY [31] with the aid of microdissection techniques demonstrated a patchy distribution of necrotic tubular lesions throughout the nephrons in the ischemic kidney. However, today there is increasing awareness of the apparent discrepancy between the physiologic alterations such as anuria or oliguria and the lack of significant histopathologic findings to support the time-honored concept of tubular necrosis as the pathogenetic lesion of acute renal failure. Recently, OLSEN and SKJOLD-BORG [32] emphasized this problem in an ultrastructural study of acute

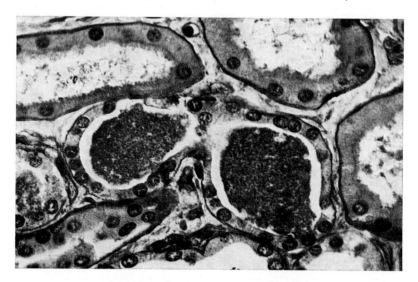

Fig. 5. Light micrograph of kidney tissue obtained at autopsy in *Case 7.* A distal tubule is filled with a typical pigmented granular cast. The tubule itself is unaltered as are several surrounding proximal tubules. Periodic acid-Schiff stain, × 1,450.

anuria associated with a variety of clinical problems including traumatic injuries and complications after surgical and obstetrical procedures. Only minimal degenerative changes in distal tubules of 10 patients with acute anuria were observed, while frank epithelial cell necrosis was extremely rare.

The most consistent renal findings were the presence of pigmented casts (fig. 5) in distal tubules, collecting ducts, and thin limbs, often associated with flattening of contiguous tubular epithelial cells, marked congestion of peritubular vessels, and mild inflammatory reaction and interstitial edema in the medulla. The exact composition of the numerous pigmented casts observed in all 5 patients remains in doubt. However, kidney sections from 4 of the patients were studied with the Pickworth stain. Variable numbers of pigmented casts were positive in all 4 kidneys studied. This finding suggests that many of the casts did contain benzidine-reactive material that presumably represented some form of heme pigment.

Etiologic Factors

Dehydration, vascular collapse, hyperpyrexia, and pigmenturia are probably factors in the production of the acute renal failure of heat stress and exercise, and, certainly, other factors such as the use of vasopressors, diminished glomerular filtration rates, and renal ischemia may be important. Dehydration has been shown to be an important component of experimentally induced renal failure [33]. Evidence of hemoconcentration was detected in 7 of the 8 patients in the present series on arrival at the hospital. Such a high incidence of hemoconcentration has not been previously reported in large series of heatstroke cases in civilian [5, 6] or military populations [3]; however, the occurrence of acute renal failure in these series was also extremely rare. This difference might suggest that the hemoconcentration in the present cases was a significant predisposing factor in the occurrence of the renal failure.

Although vascular collapse has been an accepted etiology for the acute renal failure with heatstroke [18], 2 patients in the present series had no history of hypotensive episodes. Transient unrecognized periods of hypotension sufficient to cause acute renal failure cannot be excluded, but KEW et al. [22] also did not find vascular collapse in their cases of heatstroke and renal injury. Although the policy of rapid cooling in the miners may have obscured brief periods of hypotension, the authors interpreted their results as evidence of heat-induced renal damage. This explanation would seem tenable since thermal damage has been demonstrated to occur in various mammalian tissues including renal cortex [34]. However, as with vascular collapse, acute renal failure with heat stress may occur without associated hyperpyrexia. 2 patients in the present series did not have significant temperature elevations. While hypotension, hyperpyrexia, and dehydration might all play varying roles in the renal damage after heat stress and physical exercise, pigmenturia is another possible factor. Muscle damage comparable to that which occurred in the present group was also noted by VERTEL and KNOCHEL [17] in 4 of 10 cases of acute renal failure associated with heat stress and exercise. While the authors implicated myoglobinuria in these 4 cases, the evidence was circumstantial in 3 of the cases, that is, rhabdomyolysis with dark urine. In the 4th case, spectrophotometric analysis of urine pigment was undertaken and myoglobin identified. Since the myoglobin and the hemoglobin peaks of maximal absorption are very close, conclusive separation by spectrophotometric analysis is very difficult unless the heme proteins have been converted to the carboxy derivative [35]. In the present study, the urine of one patient with dark urine, muscle damage, and renal failure was analyzed on 2 occasions by the ammonium sulfate method and was negative for myoglobin but positive for hemoglobin. Falsely negative examinations may, however, occur with this method, and a possible basis may be the existence of less soluble myoglobins, such as those separated by PERKOFF [36]. Single episodes of myoglobinuria may occur after exercise in the absence of observable heat illness and unassociated with renal failure. Nevertheless, the element of exercise and pigmenturia may be a significant factor in the present cases of acute renal failure in military recruits and may thus explain the apparent low incidence of renal failure associated with heatstroke in the nonexercising civilian population. Certainly, further study is needed to clarify this question.

Summary

Eight patients with acute renal failure associated with heat stress and physical exercise were treated at Walter Reed General Hospital between 1960 and 1966. All of the cases occurred during the summer in recruits participating in their initial 2 months of basic training.

Several unique features of the clinical course were hypercatabolism, muscle damage, prolonged periods of anuria, wide-spread system involvement, and persistent fevers without evidence of infection. Hypercatabolism was evidenced by the need for frequent and sometimes continuous peritoneal dialyses and cation-exchange resins to control the azotemia and the hyper-kalemia. Diffuse muscle involvement was found histologically in 3 fatal cases, including vacuolization, degeneration, and extensive rhabdomyolysis. Elevated serum enzymes including aldolase, serum glutamic-oxaloacetic trans-aminase, and lactic dehydrogenase that occurred concomitantly with normal liver function tests also suggested diffuse muscle involvement. Prolonged periods of anuria in 5 of the 8 cases were another prominent characteristic of the acute renal failure associated with heat stress and physical exertion. In all 5 patients postrenal obstruction was excluded as a cause of anuria by retrograde pyelography or *post-mortem* examination, and neither persistent hypotension nor dehydration could be implicated. Central nervous system, hematological, hepatic, cardiovascular, and gastrointestinal complications were also associated with the acute renal failure and made management more difficult.

The renal pathological findings revealed enlarged kidneys without histological evidence of glomerular alterations or tubular necrosis. These findings emphasized the discrepancy between the physiological alterations and the histopathological abnormalities. The most consistent findings were pigmented casts in the lumina of the distal tubules, the collecting ducts, and the thin limbs of the loops of Henle.

Dehydration, vascular collapse, hyperpyrexia, and pigmenturia (myo-globinuria or hemoglobinuria or both) were all considered to play varying etiological roles in these cases of acute renal failure associated with heat stress and exercise.

Addendum

Since completion of the present study, a 19-year-old white recruit training in South Carolina suffered acute renal failure after a 16-mile hike in an 80°F temperature and was transferred to Walter Reed General Hospital. Several features of this recent case deserve mention. Although the circumstances of the renal failure were similar to those of the other 8 cases, this patient had lived in Atlanta, Ga., before induction and is the only case of renal failure that occurred during the winter months. The onset of the illness was typical, with muscle cramps, confusion, collapse, hyperpyrexia (108°F), and hypotension, but this patient also had carpopedal spasms. An initial dark urine was positive for both hemoglobin and myoglobin (ammonium sulfate test), and muscle damage was documented with muscle biopsy, electromyography, and elevated SGOT and LDH. Complications included hyperkalemia requiring exchange resins, hypertension, and acute pulmonary edema during volume replacement. The course of the renal failure was unusual in that oliguria never intervened and dialysis was not necessary. During the initial week of the illness the patient's 24-h urine volumes ranged from 670 to 1,740 ml, while the BUN increased from 20 to 90 mg/100 ml and the creatinine increased to 8.0 mg/100 ml. Diuresis began on the 9th hospital day with subsequent return of normal renal function. None of the previous 8 patients exhibited this form of nonoliguric renal failure, but it was described in the South African gold miners.

References

1   WILLCOX, W. H.: The nature, prevention and treatment of heat hyperpyrexia: the clinical aspect. Brit. med. J. *i:* 392 (1920).

2   MORTON, T. C.: Heat effects in British service personnel in Iraq. Trans. roy. Soc. trop. Med. Hyg. *37:* 347 (1944).

3   MALAMUD, N.; HAYMAKER, W.; CUSTER, R. P.: Heat stroke: a clinico-pathological study of 125 fatal cases. Milit. Med. *99:* 397 (1946).

4   GAUSS, H. and MEYER, K. A.: Heat stroke: report of 158 cases from Cook County Hospital, Chicago. Amer. J. med. Sci. *154:* 554 (1917).

5   FERRIS, E. B.; BLANKENHORN, M. A.; ROBINSON, H. W. and CULLEN, G. E.: Heat stroke: clinical and chemical observations on 44 cases. J. clin. Invest. *17:* 249 (1938).

6   AUSTIN, M. G. and BERRY, J. W.: Observations on 100 cases of heatstroke. JAMA = J. amer. med. Ass. *161:* 1525 (1956).

7   FERGUSON, M. and O'BRIEN, M. M.: Heat stroke in New York City. Experience with twenty-five cases. N. Y. J. Med. *60:* 2531 (1960).

8   LEITHEAD, C. S.; GUTHRIE, J.; DE LA PLACE, S. and MAEGRAITH, B. G.: Incidence etiology and prevention of heat illness on ships in the Persian Gulf. Lancet *ii:* 109 (1958).

9   BARRY, M. E. and KING, B. A.: Heatstroke. Sth afr. med. J. *36:* 455 (1962).

10 EL HALAWANI, A. W.: Heat illness. I. Heat illness during the Mecca pilgrimage. WHO Chron. *18:* 283 (1964).

11 PAPADOPOULOS, N. M. and KINTZIOS, J. A.: Quantitative electrophoretic determination of lactate dehydrogenase isoenzymes. Amer. J. clin. Path. *47:* 96 (1967).

12 BERGMEYER, H. U. (ed.): Methods of enzymatic analysis, 2nd ed., p. 266 (Academic Press, New York and London 1965).

13 BERGMEYER, H. U. (ed.): Methods of enzymatic analysis, 2nd ed., p. 728 (Academic Press, New York/London 1965).

14 BLONDHEIM, S. H.: MARGOLIASH, E. and SHAFRIR, E.: A simple test for myohemoglobinuria (myoglobinuria). JAMA = J. amer. med. Ass. *167:* 453 (1957).

15 PEARCE, A. G. E. (ed.): Histochemistry, p. 928 (Little and Brown, Boston 1961).

16 McARDLE, B.: Myopathy due to a defect in muscle glycogen breakdown. Clin. Sci. *10:* 13 (1951).

17 VERTEL, R. M. and KNOCHEL, J. P.: Acute renal failure due to heat injury: an analysis of ten cases associated with a high incidence of myoglobinuria. Amer. J. Med. *43:* 435 (1967).

18 LEITHEAD, C. S. and LIND, A. R.: Heat stress and heat disorders, p. 253 (Cassell, London 1964).

19 MARCHARD, W. E. and REIMER, D.: Intravenous procaine hydrochloride in the treatment of acute renal insufficiency following heat stroke: case report. Milit. Med. *105:* 475 (1949).

20 BAXTER, C. R. and TESCHAN, P. E.: Atypical heat stroke with hypernatremia, acute renal failure, and fulminating potassium intoxication. Arch. intern. Med. *101:* 1040 (1958).

21 KNOCHEL, J. P.; BEISEL, W. R.; HERNDON, E. G., JR.; GERARD, E. S. and BARRY, K. G.: The renal, cardiovascular, hematologic and serum electrolyte abnormalities of heat stroke. Amer. J. Med. *30:* 299 (1961).

22 KEW, M. C.; ABRAHAMS, C.; LEVIN, N. W.; RUBINSTEIN, A. H. and SEFTEL, M. C.: The effects of heatstroke on renal structure and function (abstract). 3rd Int. Congr. of Nephrology, Washington, D. C., 1966, p. 220.

23 TESCHAN, P. E.; POST, R. S.; SMITH, L. H.; ABERNATHY, R. S.; DAVIS, J. H.; GRAY, D. M.; HOWARD, J. M.; JOHNSON, K. E.; KLOPP, E.; MUNDY, R. L.; O'MEARA, M. P. and RUSH, B. F., JR.: Post-traumatic renal insufficiency in military casualties I. Clinical characteristics. Amer. J. Med. *18:* 172 (1955).

24 ROMEO, J. A.: Heatstroke. Milit. Med. *131:* 669 (1966).

25 SWANN, R. C. and MERRILL, J. P.: The clinical course of acute renal failure. Medicine, Balt. *32:* 215 (1953).

26 LOUGHRIDGE, L. W.; MILNE, M. D., SHACKMAN, R., and WOOTTON, I. D. P.: Clinical course of uncomplicated acute tubular necrosis. Lancet *i:* 351 (1960).

27 SOBEL, S.; JOHNSON, W. C.; MCPHAUL, J.; MCINTOSH, D. A.; MILLER, W. E., JR., and RHOADES, E. R.: Renal mechanism in heatstroke (abstract). Clin. Res. *11:* 252 (1963).

28 OSAWA, G.; KIMMELSTIEL, P., and SEILING, V.: Thickness of glomerular basement membranes. Amer. J. clin. Path. *45:* 7 (1966).

29 JORGENSEN, F.: The ultrastructure of the normal human glomerulus. (Munksgaard, Copenhagen 1966).

30 LUCKE, B.: Lower nephron nephrosis. Milit. Med. *99:* 371 (1946).

31 OLIVER, J.; MACDOWELL, M., and TRACEY, A: The pathogenesis of acute renal failure associated with traumatic and toxic injury. Renal ischemia, nephrotoxic damage and the ischemuric episode. J. clin. Invest. *30:* 1307 (1951).

32 OLSEN, S. and SKJOLDBORG, H.: Ultrastructure of the kidney in acute anuria (abstract) 3rd Int. Congr. of Nephrology, Washington, D. C., 1966, p. 250.

33 LALICH, J.: The influence of injections of homologous hemoglobin on the kidneys of normal and dehydrated animals. J. exp. Med. *86:* 153 (1947).

34 BURGER, F. J. and FUHRMAN, F. A.: Evidence of injury by heat in mammalian tissues. Amer. J. Physiol. *206:* 1057 (1964).

35 DUMA, R. J.; TRIGG, J. W., and HAMMACK, W. J.: Primary myoglobinuria. A case report emphasizing recent diagnostic techniques. Ann. intern. Med. *56:* 97 (1962).

36 PERKOFF, G. T.: Evidence for a specific human fetal muscle heme protein. J. Lab. clin. Med. *67:* 585 (1966).

Authors' addresses: Dr. R. W. SCHRIER, Department of Medicine, University of California, San Francisco Medical Center, *San Francisco, CA 94941*; Dr. H. S. HENDERSON, Department of Medicine, University of Tennessee, *Knoxville, TN*; Dr. C. C. TISHER, Department of Medicine, Duke University School of Medicine, *Durham, NC*; Dr. R. L. TANNEN, Department of Medicine, University of Vermont Medical School, *Burlington, VT* (USA)

Medicine and Sport, vol. 5: Exercise and Cardiac Death, pp. 148–149
(Karger, Basel 1971)

Sudden Death During Exercise Due to Congenital Anomaly of Aortic Valve

E. JOKL

A 16-year-old girl collapsed and died during a dance. Autopsy revealed the presence of a congenital subaortic stenosis, an open ductus arteriosus, and extreme hypertrophy of both ventricles (fig. 1). The arrow in figure 1

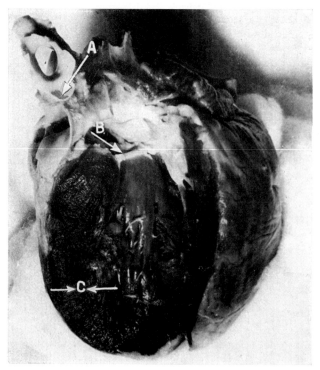

Fig. 1.

marked 'B' points to the stenotic lesion which appeared as a firm raised fibrous ring of tissue 5 mm below the base of the aortic valve. It was 4 mm in width and extended into the ventricular cavity. On microscopic examination the ring was found to be hyalinized connective tissue covered with intact flattened endothelium. With Weigert's stain the fibrous tissue was shown to contain elastic fibers. Up to the fatal seizure, there had been no signs or symptoms of the threatening catastrophe.

Though the condition is rare, a number of cases of sudden death due to it have been reported. YOUNG [1944] held that persons in whom the disease is diagnosed *in vivo* should be rejected from military service.

References

JOKL, E.: The clinical physiology of physical fitness and rehabilitation, pp. 26–27 (Thomas, Springfield 1958).

YOUNG, D.: Congenital subaortic stenosis. Amer. heart J. *28:* 440 (1944).

Author's address: University of Kentucky, *Lexington, KY 40506* (USA)

Medicine and Sport, vol. 5: Exercise and Cardiac Death, pp. 150–152
(Karger, Basel 1971)

Sudden Death of Young Athlete from Rupture of Ascending Aorta

E. Jokl and R. H. Mackintosh

A well-built athlete, aged 15, returned from a gymnastic class during which he had indulged in weight-lifting and wrestling. On reaching home he collapsed with a vice-like pain in the chest and died within 1 h.

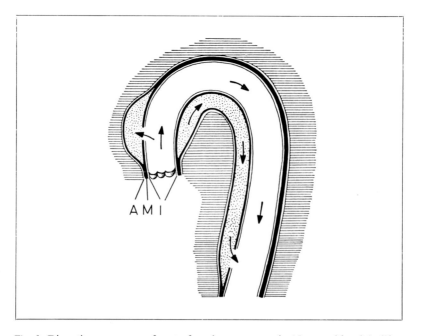

Fig. 1. Dissecting aneurysm of aorta found *post-mortem* in 15-year-old weight lifter who died after training session. A tear in the ascending aorta involving intima and media caused blood to accumulate under pressure beneath adventitia and re-entering descending aorta through second tear below.

Necropsy findings

The young man was 5 ft 8 in tall and weighed 141 lb. His musculature was strong and general development good; sexually he was retarded.

Heart. The pericardium was tense and bluish and contained 150 ml of coagulated blood and 650 ml of fluid blood and hemorrhagic serum. The left ventricle was dilated and hypertrophied, being twice the normal size. No fibrous patches were noted in the myocardium. The foramen ovale was closed. All 3 cusps of the aortic valves were present. The ductus arteriosus was patent and filled with a fresh thrombus.

Aorta. The isthmus of the aorta was so narrow that it admitted only a fine metal sound. Above the stenotic part the aorta was considerably dilated, forming a flaccid aneurysmal bag which bulged towards the right side. There was a tear 3 cm long in the lateral wall of this bag, starting just above the aortic valves and establishing a communication between the lumen of the aorta and the pericardium. The internal mammary arteries were much enlarged, their calibre corresponding to that of radial arteries of normal adult males. Below the stenosis the aorta was about half the normal width. Its walls were abnormally thin. No arteriosclerosis or atheroma was noted.

Lymphatic tissue. A persistent thymus gland, weighing 38.4 g, with active Hassall's corpuscles was found. There was an abundance of lymphatic tissue, especially in the spleen and the mesentery. Large plaques were noted in the mucosa of the small intestine.

Discussion

This case was characterised by the presence of multiple congenital anomalies of the cardiovascular system, of which the stenosis of the isthmus of the aorta is the most important. This stenosis formed a mechanical obstruction, which explains the considerable dilatation of the aorta above the isthmus, the compensatory overdevelopment of the internal mammary arteries, and the hypertrophy of the left ventricle. There were present a persistent thymus gland with active Hassall's corpuscles, hypoplastic thin-walled arteries, and a general abundance of lymphatic tissue. The immediate cause of death was rupture of the ascending aorta.

The deceased had been a first-class athlete and, though he was sexually underdeveloped, neither his general bodily growth nor his physical efficiency had been retarded by the congenital disease which caused his premature death. This observation, however, is not unique. BONNET [1903] has pointed out that, in the presence of isthmus stenosis, collateral circulation may completely compensate for the central defect. HART [1920] has published a case of sudden death in a man, aged 41, who before his fatal collapse could do strenuous physical labour. Necropsy revealed complete obliteration of the isthmus, thrombo-endocarditis of a two-cusped aortic valve, mesaortitis syphilitica of the thoracic portion of the aorta, and hypertrophy of the left ventricle. Above the obliterated isthmus the aorta showed a 'balloon-like' enlargement.

The question arises as to what part the weight-lifting and wrestling played in causing the fatal tear of the aorta. The physiological rise in blood-pressure invariably accompanying activities of this kind may have exerted a deleterious influence [JOKL, 1947].

A similar observation was reported by WASASTJERNA [1903] concerning a boy, aged 13, who collapsed while skating. JORES [1924] emphasised the general significance of physical effort in cases of rupture of the aorta in persons with stenosis of the aortic isthmus and ventricular hypertrophy. He said that, provided a good collateral circulation was established, exercise would not cause a rupture unless there was aneurysmal enlargement of the aorta and abnormal thinness of the artery walls. Contrary to what may be expected, arteriosclerosis is usually not present in cases of this kind, though the elastic elements of the artery walls are as a rule affected.

The condition is rare; among 5000 necropsies conducted between 1900 and 1905 by the Vienna Medico-Legal Institute, only 4 instances of advanced stenosis of the aortic isthmus were encountered. A good general discussion of this question can be found in the textbook of HENKE and LUBARSCH [1924].

References

BONNET, L. M.: Rev. méd. Path. *23:* 108 (1903).
HART, C.: Med. Klin. *16:* 1337 (1920).
HENKE, F. and LUBARSCH, O.: Handbuch der speziellen pathologischen Anatomie und Histologie, vol. *ii*, p. 1159 (Springer, Berlin 1924).
JOKL, E.: Syncope in athletes (Monograph, Pretoria 1947).
JORES, L.: See HENKE and LUBARSCH (1924).
WASASTJERNA, E.: Z. klin. Med. *49:* 405 (1903).

Authors' address: University of Kentucky, *Lexington, KY 40506* (USA)

Medicine and Sport, vol. 5: Exercise and Cardiac Death, pp. 153–153
(Karger, Basel 1971)

Sudden Death of a Rugby International after a Test Game

E. Jokl and E. H. Cluver

Case Report

After having played a strenuous game at Johannesburg in July, 1940, S. C. L., 32 years of age, captain of the Transvaal Representative Rugby Team, collapsed and died.

Autopsy. The body was that of an adult, European male, and was well built and muscular. Weight was 169 lb; height, 6 ft. There was marked cyanosis of the face, neck, shoulders, and fingernails. No gross abnormalities of the central nervous system were detected. There were congestion of the vessels of the brain and marked engorgement of the veins on the surface.

Significant pathologic changes were found in the circulatory system. The heart was generally hypertrophied, and weighed 482 g (17 oz). The hypertrophy was most apparent in the left ventricle, the wall of which measured 2.7 cm in thickness. There was dilatation of all of the cavities of the heart, especially of the right ventricle, which also showed hypertrophy. Its wall was 0.7 cm thick. The papillary muscles were markedly thickened and prominent. Macroscopically, the myocardium appeared firm. However, numerous *fibrotic patches* were irregulary distributed in the left ventricle. The aortic valve was competent, although the cusps were slightly thickened. The mitral valve, which was also competent, admitted 2 fingers. On the surface of the mitral valve there was a large atheromatous patch.

The entire coronary artery was underdeveloped. The left coronary artery showed *numerous atheromatous areas* which had caused marked narrowing of the lumen at 3 places. One of these *atheromatous areas* was located at the orifice of the *left coronary artery*, and another at a point about midway along the anterior descending branch. Atheromatous patches were also present in the right coronary artery. *The diameter of the ascending aorta and the aortic arch was normal, but the wall was extraordinarily soft and thin. The descending aorta measured a little over half an inch in diameter, which is less than half the normal size.* There were many atheromatous patches in various parts of the intima.

There was congestion of the thoracic and abdominal organs. The trachea and bronchi contained thick mucos. The lungs were slightly emphysematous and showed some edema and a slight excess of pigmentation. The hilar nodes were considerably enlarged.

The liver was congested, but otherwise normal; it weighed 2,495 g (5½ lb). There was considerable congestion of the spleen, and it was enlarged (weight, 454 g); on section it showed a marked excess of lymphoid tissue.

The left kidney was very small (weight, 62 g), and was the seat of advanced hydronephrosis. The parenchyma was stretched and thinned, and the pelvis was much dilated. The left ureter was sharply kinked about 1 inch above the bladder. The right kidney was greatly hypertrophied (weight, 330 g).

There was a persistent thymus gland which weighed 26 g (normal weight at this age, 15 g, according to WOLF [1] and COWDRY [2]). The genital organs were conspicuously small.

Microscopic examination. There were several areas of fibrosis in the heart muscle. The papillary muscles and the base of the left ventricle were especially affected. Areas of narrowing of the coronary arteries showed marked atheromatous thickening. The intima was greatly distorted. Atheromatous changes were also found in the aorta. The thymus gland contained scattered foci of entirely normal thymus tissue embedded in fatty tissue; there were areas of considerable infiltration and several large collections of lymphocytes. Numerous Hassall's corpuscles of large size were observed. The blood supply of the gland was abundant. The entire picture was that of an active gland, rather than the involutionary structure which one would expect at the age of 32 years [3]. Sections of the left kidney revealed normal tissue, although there was extreme congestion. The right kidney showed chronic pyelitis, fibrous thickening of the capsule, patchy fibrosis, and infiltration of the parenchyma with small round cells. All lymphoid structures were hyperplastic, including those of the throat, nasopharynx, intestinal canal, and the lymph nodes.

Previous history. L. had been one of the most prominent South African rugby players of the preceding decade. He was known as 'the iron man of rugby.' He had represented his country on the playing fields of South Africa, Britain, Australia, and New Zealand. His identical twin brother J. also died during exertion at the age of 30 years. J. was bathing in the wather at the coast when he suddenly collapsed and was swept away. The following information was kindly supplied by Major Danie Craven, captain of the Springbok team:

'I have known L. since 1931, and played on the same team with him on numerous occasions. During 1937 and 1938, I traveled with him to Australia and New Zealand, and roomed with him at various places. I always regarded L. as a very ill man. He used to complain of severe pain in the lower portion of this back. This pain he thought was due to kidney trouble. On many occasions I had to massage his back because of these pains. He also suffered from boils. After every football match he felt sick. He used to put his finger into his throat until he vomited, after which he felt better. He could not take any alcoholic drinks because they also made him sick. His stamina was exceptionally good. However, in the course of the Australia-New Zealand tour, 2 years prior to his death, his efficiency deteriorated greatly. During the last matches of the tour his performance was very poor. His strength remained outstanding, and on the boat he performed wrestling matches with the strongest of this teammates. He always had a husky voice, and suffered from chronic bronchitis. When he was tired, as, for example, after a game, he breathed heavily and noisily. He smoked at least thirty cigarettes a day.

'His twin brother J., whom I also knew very well, was apparently an identical twin. J. looked the same as L., had the same husky voice, and played the same type of game as his brother. In 1937, J. went swimming at Port Elizabeth inside the fenced portion of the beach. It was a quiet day and the water looked like a lake. After a few minutes of bathing, J. suddenly collapsed and sank. His body was never found.'

Very little information is available concerning L.'s condition immediately prior to his death. It could be ascertained, however, that, between February and July, 1940, he lost more than 20 lb in weight. This may have indicated failing health. A roentgenogram of his chest which was taken a few months before he died (anteroposterior; distance, 5 ft; standing) does not show as much cardiac hypertrophy as was present at autopsy. No lateral roentgenogram was made.

Discussion

This is a case in which a congenital developmental abnormality caused a fatal circulatory crisis in a first-class athlete. There are many remarkable features. First of all, the deceased's twin brother had died 2 years before, also during exertion. Unfortunately, *post-mortem* examination in this instance was not possible; otherwise it is more than likely that an attempt could have been made to prevent the second catastrophe. Second, study of this case emphasizes the truth of the statement made on previous occasions [4, 5] that even an extraordinarily high standard of physical efficiency is not at all a reliable indicator of the state of health of the athlete concerned. The outstanding performances of L. were possible in spite of a grossly abnormal circulatory system.

The probable development of the disease and mechanism of death may be as follows:

Development of disease. Persistence of the thymus gland arrested the normal puberty and postpuberty development of the circulatory system. This arrest of growth, which also affected the urogenital system, caused coronaries and aorta to remain in an infantile state. Consequently, the heart was compelled to pump against a greatly increased resistance. It may be assumed that the arterial blood pressure was high. Hypertrophy and dilatation of the heart followed. The lymphatic tissue throughout the body was more active than usual and the spleen was greatly enlarged.

The early development of atheromatosis can be interpreted as a result of the extraordinary hydrodynamic strain upon blood vessel walls, a strain which, under the pathologic circumstances, was aggravated by strenuous physical activities.

The heart had to work under most unfavorable conditions, and the multiple fibrotic patches in the myocardium bear witness to the deficiencies of blood supply. It is remarkable that, with such a circulatory system, the man had

been capable of such outstanding physical performances. As similar observations have been communicated by us [4-6] on several previous occasions,
it may now be accepted as an established fact that there is no strict relationship between heart disease and even outstandingly high exercise tolerance.

Mechanism of death. The mechanism of death in this case seems clear.
The deceased had taken part in a strenuous game. The oxygen requirements
of his heart were thus greatly increased. After the game he took a hot bath.
This must have shifted large amounts of blood from the intestinal circulation
into the skin. In combination with the physiologic fall of blood pressure after
the exercise, this must have added to the existing deficiency of blood supply
to the coronary artery. The significance of such physiologic phases in the
causation of the final collapse of a diseased circulation has recently been
demonstrated by BLUMGART, SCHLESINGER, and DAVIS [7]. Furthermore,
we have evidence that there were accumulation and stasis of inflammatory
exudate in the hydronephrotic right kidney, which caused contractions of
the smooth muscle of the renal pelvis and ureter. It is probable that unphys-
iologic tension in intestinal cavities elicits, by means of a reflex, spastic
contraction of the coronary arteries. This has been proved conclusively for
the stomach [8]. The autopsy also revealed signs of infection of the respiratory tract. This must have caused a further impairment of the functional
efficiency of the heart.

In 1844, ROKITANSKY [9] drew attention to the simultaneous occurrence
in adults of an infantile aorta, hypertrophy of the heart, and underdevelopment of the genital system. Although it has been assumed for a long time
that the thymus gland exerts a direct influence on puberty and postpuberty
development, it is only now that a more detailed picture can be drawn.
We are especially indebted to TIMME, whose studies made possible a full
understanding of the condition known as status thymicolymphaticus.
TIMME showed that the effects of persistence of the thymus gland, leading to
arrest of development, mostly at puberty, are often compensated by hyper-
function of other glands in the body. The primary abnormalities caused
by thymic persistence are lymphoid hyperplasia, gonadal and adrenal
deficiency, a low blood sugar level, low blood pressure, and hypoplasia of
the heart and vessels. In most cases, marked compensatory efforts of the
organism lead after some time to a profound change in the picture.

The suprarenal cortex and the pituitary are strongly stimulated. We
have asked ourselves whether the high standard of physical efficiency of
this rugby player could perhaps be explained partly by a special compensatory effort of the suprarenal cortex. The changes in the heart were

clearly the result of an attempt on the part of the circulatory system to overcome the obstacle created by the underdevelopment of the aorta.

WOLF [1] states that one of the 3 possible causes of death in cases of status thymicolymphaticus is weakness of the muscular coat of the arteries which render them incapable of withstanding sudden changes in blood pressure. This would apply in our case.

In view of the circumstances under which the sudden death of L. and his twin brother occurred, WOLF'S suggestion that swimming and bathing should be forbidden to people suffering from status thymicolymphaticus appears to be well founded.

Summary

Summarizing, it appears that death occured because of sudden coronary insufficiency. There was narrowing of the underdeveloped coronary artery caused by atheromatosis. There was the physiologic fall of blood pressure after the exercise. Large amounts of blood were shifted into the skin as a result of taking a hot bath. The oxygen requirements of the heart muscle were greatly increased through the exercise. It is probable that reflex spasm of the coronary artery was caused by the frustrated efforts of the diseased right kidney to expel its inflammatory contents. It may be assumed that permeability of the myocardial cell membranes was adversely affected by the concurrent infection of the respiratory system.

This observation allows a detailed analysis of a case of status thymico-lymphaticus, a term which has in the past often been used in a rather general way. We can trace the history of the patient back to the persistence of the thymus gland after puberty. We can thus understand the arresting effect of this primary developmental disturbance upon the maturation of the descending aorta. This latter anatomic deficiency explains the secondary pathologic reactions which created the above described extraordinary situation and caused death.

References

1   WOLF, W.: Endocrinology in modern practice. (Philadelphia and London 1939).
2   COWDRY, E. V.: Problems of ageing; in Biological and medical aspects. (London 1939). — Textbook of Histology (London 1938).

3   ASCHOFF, L.: Pathologische Anatomie, vol. 2, p. 173 (Schridde, Thymus, Jena 1923).
4   JOKL, E. and MELZER, L.: Acute fatal non-traumatic collapse during work and sport. Sth afr. J. med. Sci. *5:* 4 (1940).
5   JOKL, E.: Zusammenbrüche beim Sport (Manz, Vienna 1935).
6   JOKL, E. and PARADE: Zur Frage der Beurteilung von Herzfällen in der Sportärztlichen Praxis. Med. Klin. *32:* (1933).
7   BLUMGART, H. L.; SCHLESINGER, M. J., and DAVIS, D.: Studies on the relation of the clinical manifestations of angina pectoris, coronary thrombosis, and myocardial infarction to the pathologic findings. Amer. Heart J. *19:* 1 (1940).
8   BERGMANN, E.v.: Funktionelle Pathologie, p. 113 (Springer, Berlin 1936).
9   ROKITANSKY, C.: Handbuch der allgemeinen pathologischen Anatomie, vol. 2, p. 585 (Braumüllen und Seidel, Wien 1844).

Authors' address: University of Kentucky, *Lexington, KY 40506* (USA)

Medicine and Sport, vol. 5: Exercise and Cardiac Death, pp. 159–165
(Karger, Basel 1971)

Myocardial Infarction in Twenty-Year-Old Identical Twins

F. L. Giknis, D. E. Holt, H. W. Whiteman, M. D. Singh,
A. Benchimol and E. G. Dimond

Twin studies provide valuable information for assessment of genetic factors involved in a disease process. There have been relatively few studies reported using clinical coronary artery disease as the trait [1–4], and these, in general, support the hypothesis of a significant genetic factor [5].

This report documents myocardial infarctions in 20-year-old identical twins, probably occurring at about the same time.

Case Reports

The identical twins, T. C. and T. O. C., were 20-year-old Caucasian males of Northern European ancestry born and reared in Georgia. The paternal grandfather died of heart disease in the seventh decade, and a paternal uncle was suspected of having some nonfatal type of cardiac disorder. The family history was otherwise negative for heart disease. The father had undergone surgical treatment for peptic ulcer. The mother and two younger siblings were well.

Past histories were unremarkable. The twins had tonsillectomies at the same time in childhood. There were no serious illnesses and no suggestions of any type of previous cardiovascular or renal disorder. The twins had put on boxing exhibitions in childhood, starting at age six years. They were athletically inclined, and their physical conditions were considered excellent. Their diets were average American, save that milk, butter and eggs were favored and possibly consumed in greater than average quantities. Occupational histories revealed no known exposure to noxious agents. T. C. appeared to be his father's favorite. T. O. C.'s relationships with the father were occasionally stressful. Despite this, T. C. joined the Navy at age 17 years, while T. O. C. remained at home.

T. C.'s naval career was not complicated by promotions. In September 1961 he was thrown from a horse and hospitalized for treatment of bilateral Colles' fracture. No cardiac abnormality was noted on examination at that time. Blood pressure was normal, as was the chest film. In the summer of 1962, T. C. joined his base's boxing team. This

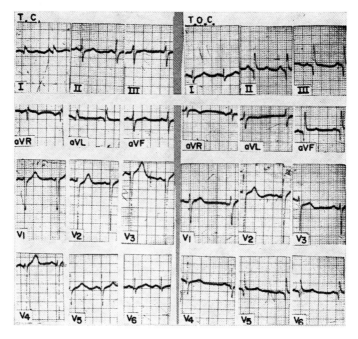

Fig. 1. Twins' ECGs, August 1963 (see text). *a:* standard and unipolar leads, *b:* precordial leads.

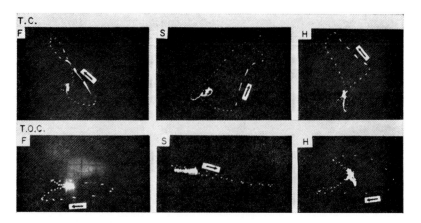

Fig. 2. Twins' vectorcardiograms, Frank system; H = horizontal, F = frontal, S = left sagittal (see text).

entailed running 4–5 miles daily, and there were 3-h gymnasium 'workouts' which he withstood without symptoms. In the fall of 1962 he noted left chest pain and tenderness after holding up a 200-lb fender. A pulled muscle was diagnosed.

Twin 1. Meanwhile, back in Georgia, T. O. C. was in his usual state of good health until May 2, 1963 when he noted onset of severe chest pain while *bowling*. This was associated with nausea and diaphoresis. He stopped bowling and remained seated for 2 h, until his symptoms subsided sufficiently so that he was able to leave the bowling alley. He awoke feeling fine after a night's rest and had no further symptoms until May 16, when chest pain recurred at work. He was admitted to a local hospital where opiates relieved his pain. Physical examination revealed no significant abnormality. Complete blood count, urinalysis, sedimentation rate and chest film were normal. The initial serum glutamic oxala-acetic transaminase determination was 52 units. The ECGs and vectorcardiogram were consistent with an inferior infarction with lateral involvement (fig. 1 and 2). His 3 weeks' hospitalization was uneventful.

Twin 2. T. C. stated that he did not know of his brother's illness when he had a sudden impulse to go home on leave, sensing that something was wrong. He arrived at home to find his brother hospitalized. He states that during this leave period, while *lifting a large pipe* in his backyard, he noted severe, constricting, anterior chest pain associated with lightheadedness, nausea, diaphoresis and dyspnea which persisted for 30 to 45 min. He did not seek medical advice, feeling that he would report this to his medical officer on return from leave. Thereafter he had recurrent chest pain with and without effort, which varied somewhat in location and character. There was associated tenderness on lying on his left side. Most of his symptoms were believed to be musculoskeletal in origin. He finally reported to his dispensary, where an ECG was taken and noted to be abnormal.

T. C. was admitted for study in September 1963. He indicated that his usual weight was 132 lb, but because of decreased physical activity he had gained a few pounds. He admitted smoking 10–15 cigarettes daily and occasionally used alcoholic beverages. Physical examination revealed a blood pressure of 120/80 mm Hg. The patient was mesomorphic in build, 67 inches in height, 135 lb in weight. Neither arcus senilis, xanthelasma nor xanthomatous lesions were present. A grade 1–2/6, short, soft, midsystolic murmur at the apex was the only notable feature on physical examination. Extensive laboratory evaluation included normal complete blood count, urinalysis, blood urea nitrogen, glucose tolerance test, serum enzymes and electrolytes. Both ECG and vectorcardiogram were suggestive of an anterolateral myocardial infarction (fig. 1 and 2), but serial records and laboratory studies indicated no evidence of an active process.

Left heart catheterization was accomplished in October 1963, retrograde via the right femoral artery. There was no gradient across the aortic valve. Left ventricular pressures were 82/3 mm Hg with an end-diastolic pressure of 14. A simultaneous apexcardiogram revealed a large A wave. *Coronary angiography* was accomplished by the flush technic with ventricular arrest. The main segment of the left coronary artery showed a medium-sized defect about 2 cm from its origin from the aorta. The left circumflex branch was totally occluded at its origin. There was retrograde flow through the left anterior descending coronary artery to the circumflex artery with a significant number of small collateral vessels around the area of the occluded vessel (fig. 3).

Studies of blood lipids carried out simultaneously revealed T. O. C. to have normal values, while T. C.'s were borderline to slightly high. Blood types were similar (table I).

The twins had been observed together (H. W. W.) and their appearance suggested that they were identical twins.

T. C. was medically discharged from the Navy. The twins were seen in May 1964. They were symptom-free and working regularly. T. O. C.'s ECG was unchanged, while T. C.'s revealed T-wave changes toward normal in the anterolateral leads (fig. 4).

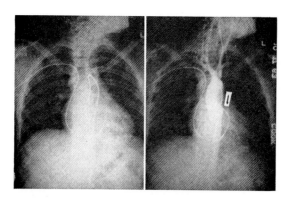

Fig. 3. Twin 2. T.C.'s coronary angiograms. *a:* scout film showing position of catheters. *b:* following injection into the aortic root. The arrow indicates the site of occlusion in the left circumflex artery. The faint trace of dye in the left circumflex is due to retrograde filling.

Table I. Twins' blood studies

	T.C.	Normal for laboratory	T.O.C.
A. Serum Lipid Studies			
Phospholipids	224	226 ± 16	214
Triglycerides	118	120 ± 30	93
Cholesterol	295	250 ± 20	240
B. Blood Typing			
ABO	A		A
Rh	Negative		Negative
Group M	Positive		Positive
Group N	Positive		Positive
Kell	Negative		Negative

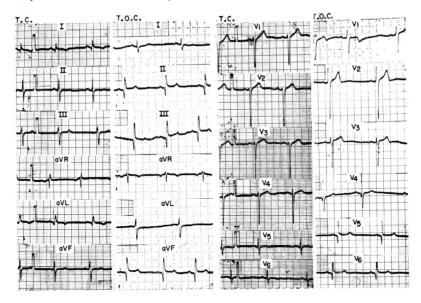

Fig. 4. Twins' follow-up ECGs, May 1964 (see text).

Comment

Though T. O. C.'s (twin 1) initial coronary occlusion may have occurred a few weeks prior to hospitalization, it could be dated with some accuracy. The electrocardiographic and vector study left little doubt as to the nature of his disease. T. C.'s (twin 2) electrocardiographic abnormalities were less striking, but his occlusion was documented by coronary artery visualization. The timing of his difficulties was less certain. He had a variety of musculo-skeletal type chest pain, but the only severe episode suggestive of angina occurred while his brother was hospitalized. The coronary angiocardiographic pattern was not inconsistent with the possibility of the occlusion occurring at this time [6], and the changes in the follow-up ECG added further support to this possibility. It was quite probable, therefore, that both infarctions occurred within the period of a few weeks.

Type of twins. On the basis of the patients' own impression, observation of the twins and the blood studies made, we have diagnosed the twins as uniovular, realizing the possibility of error. Though description of birth membranes was not available, these need not establish the type of twins with certainty. A single chorion indicates monozygosity, though many monozygotic pairs have two chorions. All that can be said is that a single placenta makes monozygosity considerably more probable, while two placentas are more likely with a dizygotic pair. Blood grouping is valuable in that a single difference in any of the groups precludes monozygosity, while identical blood types, at most, support this possibility. The most common mistake, therefore, is to class erroneously a pair of twins as monozygotic [7].

Location of infarction. A significant variable in the cases was the location of the infarction, T. C.'s being anterolateral and T. O. C.'s inferolateral. Either the site of occlusion or the pattern of dominance was, therefore, different. Angiograms proved that T. C. did not have a left dominant pattern [8], which would have had to have been the case for T. O. C., if it were assumed that the areas of occlusion were similar. Though one would anticipate similar electrocardiographic patterns in identical twins, this need not be the case. In a study of 32 sets of identical twins, 16 had close similitary, 8 pairs had some similarity and the remaining 8 pairs of twins had no similarity in their electrocardiographic patterns [9].

Serum lipid studies. There was no evidence to suggest hypercholesteremia or hyperlipemia in our subjects by history, physical examination or laboratory study. T. C.'s lipid studies were borderline high, while T. O. C.'s were normal. At the time of these determinations T. O. C. was months convalescent, while T. C. was still suspect of having coronary artery disease. While T. O. C. had time to alter his diet, T. C. had gained some weight on a diet known to be high in fats. This would support the findings of OSBORNE and ADLERSBERG [10], who noted similar serum cholesterol levels when uniovular twins were living together but some difference when they were separated. They concluded that both hereditary and environment were important in lipid studies in twins.

The demonstration of localized disease, at least in the case of T. C., raised the possibility of surgical treatment, particularly endarterectomy. In that symptoms were minimal and collateral vessels were demonstrated, this approach awaits follow-up evaluation.

Summary

Myocardial infarctions in 20-year-old identical twins are reported. Coronary angiography located the occlusion site in one of the twins. The history raises the strong possibility that both infarctions may have occurred within a period of weeks.

References

1   PARADE, G. W. and LEHMAN, W.: Angina pectoris bei erbgleichen Zwillingen. Klin. Wschr. *17:* 1036 (1938).

2   KAHLER, O. H. and WEBER, R.: Zur Erbpathologie von Herz- und Kreislauf-erkrankungen. Z. klin. Med. *137:* 507 (1939).

3   FROMENT, R.; GUINET, P.; VIGNON, G., and MARTIN-NOËL: Angor coronarien athé-romateux, à début précoce et à évolution parallèle chez deux jumeaux. Arch. mal. cœur *38:* 260 (1945).

4   BENEDICT, R. B.: Coronary heart disease in identical female twins. Amer. J. Med. *23:* 814 (1958).

5   McKUSICK, V. A.: Genetic factors in cardiovascular diseases: I. The four main types of cardiovascular disease. Mod. Conc. cardiovasc. Dis. *28:* 535 (1959).

6   LAURIE, W. and WOODS, J. D.: Anastomosis in coronary circulation. Lancet *ii:* 812 (1958).

7   ROBERTS, J. A. F.: An introduction to medical genetics, 4th ed. p. 235 (Oxford University Press, London 1963).

8   SCHLESINGER, M. J.: Relation of the anatomic pattern to pathological conditions of the coronary arteries. Arch. Path. *30:* 403 (1940).

9   WISE, N. B.; COMEAU, W. J., and WHITE, P. D.: An electrocardiographic study of twins. Amer. Heart J. *46:* 99 (1953).

10 OSBORNE, R. H. and ADLERSBERG, D.: Serum lipids in adult twins. Science *127:* 1294 (1958).

Authors' address: Dr. F. L. GIKNIS, Dr. D. E. HOLT, Dr. H. W. WHITEMAN, Dr. M. D. SINGH, Dr. A. BENCHIMOL and Dr. E. G. DIMOND, 2707 32nd Street NW, *Washington, DC* (USA)

Medicine and Sport, vol. 5: Exercise and Cardiac Death, pp. 166–175
(Karger, Basel 1971)

Sudden Unexpected Death in Three Generations

J. R. Green, L. J. Krovetz, D. R. Shanklin, J. J. DeVito, and
W. J. Taylor.

Ten instances of sudden unexpected deaths were identified in 3 generations. Average age at death was 21 years, and in one generation 30% died
abruptly at an average age of 13. Syncopal episodes heralded death in 80%,
but no other signs or symptoms of cardiovascular disease existed. No abnormalities were found in 22 members of recent generations. Serial study of
the conduction systems of 2 patients revealed minor variances from normal.
Perhaps a nonsex-linked gene has produced minor anatomical defects of
the conduction system which could predispose to the development of fatal
arrhythmias by a variety of environmental factors. The Lev technique for
bundle studies of the conduction system should be used in similar instances
of unexplained death with grossly normal hearts.

The drama of the startling death of a 15-year-old boy just as he completed a race in a school track meet was heightened by the collapse and
demise of his 14-year-old sister a few hours later on hearing of her sibling's
death. Suspicion that this was not mere coincidence was aroused when a
preliminary investigation revealed that an apparently healthy younger
sister had fainted while walking on a beach a year earlier and could not be
resuscitated from ventricular fibrillation. Accordingly, a detailed historical
survey of the 4 preceding generations of this family was made. This revealed
an unusually high incidence of unanticipated death, predominantly in a
young age group.

Sudden, unexpected death is defined as occurring in a matter of minutes
or a few hours in a person who up to the moment appeared to be in good
health. This, of course, excludes accidental death. The more common
causes of such an event are coronary artery disease, cerebral vascular
accidents, myocardiopathies, and cardiac conduction disturbances. Certain

of these disorders may have an increased familial incidence but diagnostic, clinical, and pathological findings are generally present. Anatomical studies in the present patients failed to disclose gross abnormalities. Furthermore electrocardiographic studies on 22 members of the family, including an ECG from one of the members who died suddenly, failed to show any evidence of a conduction defect.

A survey of the literature reveals that 10% of those who die of 'natural causes' do so suddenly and unexpectedly at a mean age of 50.3 years. The increased incidence in the present family and the significantly younger age of those dying makes this family decidedly different from the general population.

Anatomical variants in the conduction system of the hearts of the more recent victims suggest a theoretical cause for death.

Family history

The propositus was a 15-year-old boy who had always been in excellent health. Two weeks before his death, a thorough physical examination revealed no abnormalities. Although he had been adequately conditioned for track, he died abruptly at the end of a 100-yard sprint.

The 14-year-old sister of the lad had been examined at the Shands Teaching Hospital one year previously. Physical examination, chest roentgenogram and ECG were normal. In the past, she had experienced occasional brief syncopal episodes. When informed of her brother's death, she fainted. Sensing that this was not a usual episode, her family employed closed chest massage, assisted her respirations and rushed her to her family physician where an ECG revealed ventricular fibrillation. Efforts to resuscitate her, including electrical defibrillation, were futile.

The 10-year-old sister of these children had died suddenly and unexpectedly one year previously while playing on a beach. Prior to this event, she had been considered to be in perfect health.

Communication with the family patriarchs, the use of family Bibles and church records, investigation of recordings of the local historical societies, minutes of the local and state legislative bodies, and physician and hospital records permitted the compilation of a family history dating from the early 1800s to the present (fig. 1). The family is of predominantly French and English stock, and its members were among the founding settlers of one of the oldest communities in the United States. They have been politically active since the 1800s and are justifiably proud of their

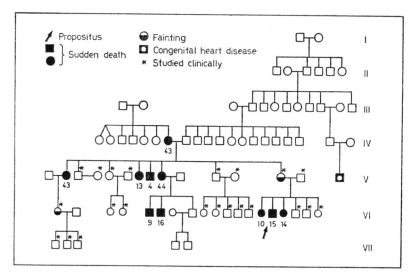

Fig. 1. Family tree from the early 1800s to present generations.

heritage, so that records of the activities and lives of the family are remarkably complete for the past 168 years.

Ten instances of sudden unexpected deaths appear in these archives. The affected members, the age at death, previous history, events immediately preceding death, and autopsy data when available are listed in table 1. Death was heralded by syncopal episodes in 80% of the victims but no other signs or symptoms of cardiovascular disease had been noted. The average age at sudden death was 21 years. Half of the members in generation V (4 of 8) died unexpectedly at an average age of 26 years, while in generation VI, an abrupt demise was the fate of 30% (5 of 17) at an average age of 13 years.

Clinical study

Twenty-two members of generations V, VI, and VII were examined. Complete medical histories and physical examinations yielded no abnormalities except for a history of fainting in member V-13 (the mother of three victims of sudden death) and in VI-1. All had normal chest roentgenograms (4 views with barium swallow), and ECGs at rest.

Since none of the deceased family members had preceding histories of disease states, or physical signs or laboratory findings indicating disease,

Table I. Ages and events of the members who died suddenly and unexpectedly [1]

Family member	Sex	Age at sudden death	Event-preceding death	Comments
IV-7	F	43	Watching a dance	Had previous fainting spells; no autopsy
V-2	F	43	Talking on a phone	Had previous fainting spells; no autopsy
V-7	F	13	On the way to a dance	Had previous fainting spells; no autopsy
V-8	M	4	During an argument	No autopsy
V-9	F	44	Trying to get into her locked home	Had previous fainting spells; no autopsy
VI-5	M	9	Playing in his yard	Had previous fainting spells; no autopsy
VI-6	M	16	Following a beach rescue as a lifeguard	Had previous fainting spells; findings of gross heart examination were normal
VI-14	F	10	Playing on a beach	Ventricular fibrillation was documented; findings of gross heart examination were normal
VI-15	M	15	At the end of a foot race	Complete autopsy
VI-16	F	14	Told of brother's death	Ventricular fibrillation was documented; had previous fainting spells; complete autopsy

1 Deaths in generation V, 50%; average age, 26. Deaths in generation VI, 30%; average age, 13.

but almost all of them had episodes of fainting prior to their death, a reasonable hypothesis was that these individuals were unusually sensitive to physical or psychic stress or both which triggered a fatal arrhythmia. If such could be defined, a pharmacological approach to therapy could be planned. Therefore, ECGs were taken during and after graded exercise to the point of strenuous work with a bicycle ergometer. Only in the 48-year-old mother of the recently deceased children was an unusual response elicited. During her first exercise test employing a workload of 25 W (comparable to bicycling on a level surface), bigeminal rhythm developed from premature ventricular contractions. Exercise was stopped and in 10 minutes her tracing was normal. Urinary catecholamines and blood electrolytes tested that day were normal. One month later when she was restudied, no abnormalities appeared in her exercise ECGs. Smoking, infusions of 1 mg of atropine sulfate intravenously, and the infusion of levarterenol bitartrate to a level of 6 μg/min and epinephrine to a level of 15 μg/min caused no change in her ECG.

Pathological study

Complete gross autopsies of the propositus (VI–15) and of his sister (VI–16) were normal. The hearts were normal in size, shape, and weight. The coronary arteries were normal and the great vessel distribution was correct.

The conduction system was studied with the use of the semiserial conduction method of LEV [1] as modified by SHANKLIN and LAITE [2]. In this method, portions of atrial and ventricular septa containing the bundle are systematically sectioned and then reconstructed yielding a 3-dimensional view of the course of the approaches, the atrioventricular node, and the bundle of His and its major branches.

The heart of the propositus (VI–15) revealed a bundle with a number of spurious blind-end branches as it passed through the pars membranacea which had no attachment or insertion to the ventricular myocardium. The hypoplastic bundle continued into the ventricular myocardium. The atrioventricular node was indistinct and the approach tissue seemed to give rise directly to the bundle of His itself. The nodal artery could not be identified. The heart of member VI–16 showed an exceedingly small and short bundle which inserted into the right myocardium before it became separated from the bifurcation. The atrioventricular node was indistinct.

Comment

The present investigation concerns 10 sudden deaths within a single family. It is estimated that among deaths in the general population, 10% are sudden and unexpected [3]. Table II presents a large series of sudden deaths in the literature [4–6] including an analysis of the references listed under the largest of these studies as a basis for statistical comparison [7–16]. Ages at death are given both for the persons where cause of death was established and also for those without identifiable cause. If these 10 individuals were random members of the general population, the probability that all their deaths would be abrupt and unanticipated would be 0.10 [10] or 1 chance in 10 billion. It is concluded that with respect to the incidence of sudden and unexpected death, this family is decidedly different from the general population.

Employing the results of the studies in table II as being representative of age at unexpected death for the population in general, the mean age at the time of death was 49.1 with a standard deviation of 15.7 years. For the 10 family members who are the basis for this study the average age at death was 21.1 years. Of course, if certain of the remaining family members die under similar circumstances, this will be altered, but probably not significantly, to influence the statistical significance. The probability that 10 deaths selected at random would have an average age of 25 years or less can be determined from the tables of the Normal or Gaussian distribution. This gives a probability of less than 1 chance in 1 million. Thus, it may be concluded that in addition to the incidence data, the family presented is decidedly different from the general population with respect to age at the time of sudden and unexpected death. These two statistical analyses confirm without question that the incidence of this type of death in this family is not due to chance.

Historically, the confirmation of sudden and unexpected death is excellent in this family. Physician reports, hospital records, and family histories corroborated this fact. The events immediately preceding death were associated with varying degrees of physical or psychic stress or both. Of those dying, 80% had previous episodes of fainting associated with psychic stresses. Although no autopsy examination was performed in 6, normal findings of gross heart examinations were present in 2, as were complete autopsy information in an additional 2 members except as described.

The most common cause of sudden death is coronary artery disease resulting in disturbances of cardiac conduction from localized myocardial

Table II

Source	Number of persons	Cause of death established	No cause of death established	Ages at death[1]										Comments
				Birth-10	10-20	20-30	30-40	40-50	50-60	60-70	70-80	80-90	90	
KULLER et al. [4]	101	100%	0	...	...	...	...	...	...	...	...	...	...	Study limited to 20-39-year-old bracket
HELPERN and RABSON [5]	2,030	100%	0	...	...	...	...	...	...	...	...	...	...	...
BURCH and DEPASQUALE [6]	8,151	98%	2%	...	...	...	...	...	...	...	...	...	...	Peak age given as 20-70 years; no ages given for 2% of deaths where no cause was identified
CAIRNS [7]	500	99.6%	0.4%	...	...	...	...	...	...	...	...	...	...	No ages given
KOPPISCH [8]	61	90%	10%	9	6	7	9	12	7	1[2]	0	1	...	No ages given in 9 instances
BEDFORD [9]	198	92%	8%[3]	6	6	5	20	28	39	60	15	1	...	No ages given in 14 instances
LAUREN [10]	403	99.3%	0.7%[3]	...	12	36	48	70	93	79	53	11	...	Birth through 15 years not studied

Source	Number of persons	Cause of death established	No cause of death established	Ages at death[1] Birth-10	10-20	20-30	30-40	40-50	50-60	60-70	70-80	80-90	90	Comments
RABSON and HELPERN [11]	2,030	100%	0	...	...	...	...	...	...	...	...	...	...	Ages given only for persons dying with coronary artery disease (45%); peak incidence of death was 44-69 years
MORITZ and ZAMCHEK [12]	Approx. 1,000	96.7%	3.3%[3]	...	...	...	...	...	...	...	...	...	...	Study of men 18-40 years; author lists 10% but pathological evidence of disease was present in 6.7%
RICHARDS [13]	200	100%	0	...	...	...	...	...	...	...	...	...	...	No ages given
JAFFE [14]	73	98.6%	1.4%	...	...	...	.	...	...	...	...	...	...	No ages given
SHELDON [15]	798	100%	0	...	...	...	...	...	...	...	...	...	...	No ages given
WEYRICH [16]	2,668	99%	0.89%[3]	...	...	...	...	...	...	...	...	...	...	Line graph was presented

1 Numbers above broken lines are for patients in whom cause of death was established; below broken lines, where cause was not established.
2 Death occurred 2 days after surgery.
3 No ages given.

ischemia or injury [17]. The young age at time of death in this family, and lack of evidence of coronary artery disease or myocardial fibrosis at autopsy, militates against this being a likely explanation.

The sudden death which is common in idiopathic myocardiopathies [18, 19] and the type of familial obstructive myocardiopathy variously described as asymmetrical hypertrophy of the heart [20], muscular subaortic stenosis [21], idiopathic hypertrophic subaortic stenosis [22], obstructive cardiomyopathy [23], and hereditary cardiovascular dysplasia [24] naturally had to be considered, since unexplained sudden death at an early age is a feature, particularly in the familial form of the disease.

Clinical studies on 22 members of this family failed to reveal signs or symptoms of congestive heart failure or cardiomegaly which are prominent features of familial myocardiopathies, nor was the distinctive pathological picture present in the members on whom autopsies were performed.

Familial cardiac conduction disturbances have been noted infrequently [25–27]. There are reports of conduction disturbances in 2 generations [28–30]. Recently a family was reported in which there were conduction disturbances in 3 generations and, by history, in the 4th generation [31]. The common feature of these reports is ECG evidence of varying degrees of atrioventricular block. Electrocardiograms of 22 members of the family described here, including one member who died suddenly, failed to show any evidence of a conduction defect.

JERVEL and LANGE-NIELSEN [32] recognized the association of deaf-mutism, fainting, and sudden death in a population of autosomal recessive inheritance. No structural heart disease was found; however, pronounced prolongation of the QT interval produced characteristic ECGs. WARD [33] described a similar or identical entity in 2 siblings with normal hearing and prolongation of the QT interval associated with attacks of syncope due to ventricular fibrillation. No QT abnormalities were present in the ECGs of the members studied in this communication including one member who died suddenly.

The detailed serial study of the conduction system in the two recent instances of sudden death revealed an absent nodal artery in one, and hypoplasia of the right bundle branch and spurious branches of the bundle of His in both. The degree to which a congenitally malformed conduction system predisposes an individual to arrhythmias is unknown. JAMES [34] recently described focal degeneration of the His bundle, which was associated with bone formation in the adjacent central fibrous body in 10 Doberman Pinscher dogs that died suddenly and unexpectedly. He hypothesized that a hereditary abnormality of the coronary arteries was responsible for the pathological findings and that this led to arrhythmia and death.

The suggestive evidence of conduction system abnormalities in the instances described and the high frequency of fainting episodes preceding death in this family suggest the hypothesis that a nonsex-linked gene has produced minor anatomical defects of the conduction system which could predispose to the development of fatal arrhythmias by a variety of environmental factors. It is urged that the LEV [1] technique for bundle studies of the conduction system from the sinus node through the distal ramifications be used in similar instances of unexplained death with grossly normal hearts.

References

1   LEV, M.; WIDRAN, J.; and ERIKSON, E. E.: A method for the histopathic study of the atrioventricular node, bundle, and branches. Arch. Path. *52:* 73–83 (1951).
2   SHANKLIN, D. R. and LAITE, M. B.: Pickett-Sommer film strip technique. Arch. Path. *75:* 91–93 (1963).
3   MORITZ, A. R.: Unexpected death of apparently healthy adults from natural causes, NW. Med. *47:* 500–503 (1948).
4   KULLER, L.; LILIENFELD, A., and FISHER, R.: Sudden and unexpected deaths in young adults: an epidemiological study. JAMA = J. amer. med. Ass. *198:* 248–252 (1966).
5   HELPERN, M. and RABSON, S. M.: Suddden and unexpectcd natural death: General considerations and statistics, N. Y. J. Med. *45:* 1197–1201 (1945).
6   BURCH, G. E. and DEPASQUALE, N. P.: Sudden unexpected natural death. Amer. J. med. Sci. *249:* 112–123 (1965).
7   CAIRNS, F. J.: Sudden and unexpected deaths. New Zeald med. J. *51:* 74–81 (1952).
8   KOPPISCH, E.: On the causes of sudden death in Puerto Rico: Analysis of 61 cases studied *post-mortem*. Puerto Rico J. publ. Hlth trop. Med. *9:* 328–345 (1934).
9   BEDFORD, T. H. B.: The pathology of sudden death. J. Path. Bact. *36:* 333–347 (1933).
10 LAUREN, E.: On sudden and unexpected death in medicolegal practice. Acta path. microbiol. scand. *14:* 40–88 (1937).
11 RABSON, S. M. and HELPERN, M.: Sudden and unexpected death: II. Coronary artery sclerosis. Amer. Heart J. *35:* 635–642 (1948).
12 MORITZ, A. R. and ZAMCHEK, N.: Sudden and unexpected deaths of young soldiers. Arch. Path. *42:* 459–494 (1946).
13 RICHARDS, R.: A note on the causation of sudden death. Brit. med. J. *ii:* 51–53 (1947).
14 JAFFE, R.: Ueber plötzliche Todesfälle und ihre Pathogenese. Dtsch. med. Wschr. *64:* 2010–2012 (1928).
15 SHELDON, S.: Sudden and uncertified deaths. Med. J. Aust. *1:* 252–256 (1932).
16 WEYRICH, G.: Erfahrungen über den plötzlichen Tod aus natürlicher Ursache bei Erwachsenen. Dtsch Z. Ges. gerichtl. Med. *18:* 211–222 (1931).

17 PRUITT, R. D.: On sudden death. Amer. Heart J. *68:* 111–118 (1964).
18 FOWLER, N. O.: Classification and differential diagnosis of the myocardiopathies Progr. cardiovasc. Dis. *7:* 1–16 (1964).
19 EVANS, W.: Familial cardiomegaly. Brit. Heart J. *11:* 68–82 (1949).
20 TEARE, D.: Asymmetrical hypertrophy of the heart in young adults. Brit. Heart J. *20:* 1–8 (1958).
21 BRENT, L. B., et al.: Familial muscular subaortic stenosis. Circulation *21:* 167–180 (1960).
22 BRAUNWALD, E., et al.: Idiopathic hypertrophic subaortic stenosis. Amer. J. Med. *29:* 924–945 (1960).
23 HOLLMAN, A., et al.: A family with obstructive cardiomyopathy (asymmetrical hypertrophy). Brit. Heart J. *22:* 449–456 (1960).
24 PARE, J. A. P., et al.: Hereditary cardiovascular dysplasia. Amer. J. Med. *31:* 37–62 (1961).
25 OSLER, W.: On the so-called Stokes-Adams disease: Slow pulse with syncopal attacks. Lancet *ii:* 516–524 (1903).
26 AYLWARD, R. D.: Congenital heart block. Brit. med. J. *i:* 943 (1928).
27 WALLGREN, G. and AGORIO, E.: Congenital complete A-V block in three siblings. Acta paediat. *49:* 49–56 (1960).
28 FULTON, Z. M. K.; JUDSON, C. F., and NORRIS, G. W.: Congenital heart block occurring in a father and two children, one an infant. Amer. J. med. Sci. *140:* 339–348 (1910).
29 WALLGREN, A. and WINBLAD, S.: Congenital heart block. Acta Paediat. *20:* 175–204 (1938).
30 WENDKOS, M. H. and STUDY, R. S.: Familial congenital A-V heart block. Amer. Heart J. *34:* 138–142 (1947).
31 GAZES, P. C., et al.: Congenital familial cardiac conduction disturbances. Circulation *32:* 32–34 (1965).
32 JERVELL, A. and LANGE-NIELSEN, F.: Congenital deaf-mutism, functional heart disease with prolongation of the QT interval, and sudden death. Amer. Heart J. *54:* 59–68 (1945).
33 WARD, O. C.: A new familial cardiac syndrome in children. J. Irish med. Ass. *54:* 103–106 (1964).
34 JAMES, T. N. and DRAKE, E. H.: Sudden death in Doberman Pinschers. Amer. J. intern. Med. *68:* 821–829 (1968).

Authors' address: Dr. J. R. GREEN, Department of Medicine, Division of Cardiology. University of Florida, College of Medicine, *Gainesville, FL 32801* (USA)

Subject Index

Accident proneness 57
Acetylsalicylic acid 58
Age 33, 63, 64, 86
Alcohol 49, 58, 60, 61
Altitude 32, 56
Amnesia 25, 43
Amphetamines 59
Analgesics 58
Anemia 88
Aneurysm 15, 19, 46, 71
Anticholinergics 61
Antihistamines 55, 58
Anuria 122
Aorta 15, 41, 45, 148, 150
Aortic aneurysm 15
Aortic regurgitation 15, 45
Aortic stenosis 41, 45
Appendicitis 47
Arteriosclerosis in children 64
Artery of Death 87
Asymptomatic disease 1
Asystole 41
Atmospheric pressure 88
Atrio-ventricular node 108
Atropine 62

Bacilluria 45
Barbiturates 58, 60
Bethesda Conference 35
Blood dyscrasias 58
Blood pressure 13
Blood urea nitrogen 123
Bromides 58
Bronchopneumonia 127
Bundle branch block 45

Candida albicans 125
Carbon monoxide 55, 88
Cardiac catheterization 72
Cardiac standstill 42
Cardiac tumors 1
Cerebellar degeneration 125
Cerebral anemia 55
Cerebral aneurysm 19
Cerebral atrophy 45
Cerebral hemorrhage 125
Cerebral tumors 44
Chest trauma 71, 77
Chlorpheniramine 56
Claudication 71
Cold 114
Collapses 23
Conduction system 103
Confusion 25, 43
Congenital anomalies 1, 91, 148
Coronary atherosclerosis 1, 32, 34
Cyanosis 23

Deaf children 108
Death from exhaustion 5
Death of wrestler 82
Decongestants 58
Digitalis 125
Drugs and flying 58

Electrical instability 42
Electrocardiogram 33, 42, 160, 163
Electroencephalogram 44
Electrophoresis 48
Emboli 78
Emotional stress 45

Endocarditis 67, 101
Epidemiology 49
Epilepsy 43, 44, 55, 57, 103
Evaluation of accidents 33
Exercise and sudden death 39
Exercise capacity 36
Exercise tolerance 85
Exhaustion and death 5
Expiratory effort 13
Extrasystoles 14, 45

Fainting 45, 55, 103
Fatal seizures 84
Fibroma of heart 3
Fitness 15
Flying personnel 25
Four Inns Walking Competition 112
Functional pathology 13

Ganglionic block 60
Gastro-coronary reflex 14, 22
Gastrointestinal hemorrhage 58
Genetics 40, 159, 166
Glucose tolerance 44

Hassal's bodies 41, 151, 154
Heartblock 14, 45, 55
Heart disease and flying 35
Heatstroke 5, 121
Hematuria 48
Hemorrhagic cyst 41
Hepatitis 134
Hydrocortison 125
Hypercholesteremia 41
Hyperpyrexia 137
Hyperuricemia 61
Hyperventilation 45
Hypoglycemia 44
Hypoplasia of arteries 19, 153
Hypoplasia of bundle 170
Hypothermia causing death 114
Hypoxia 85

Idiosyncrasies 58
Iliac emboli 15
Infection 45, 59, 86, 88, 114, 127, 134
Influenza 114
Insulin 57
Intragastric pressure 14
Intravascular thrombi 43
Ischemic heart disease 25

Jaundice 45

Kalaazar 45

Loss of blood 88

Malaria 45
Mannitol 122
Marathon running 15
Master systems of body 12, 19
Medical examination 36
Meprobamate 60
Methemoglobinemia 58
Mitral insufficiency 69
Mitral stenosis 15, 22
Motion sickness 59
Mural thrombosis 78
Muscle relaxants 61
Myocardial contusion 77
Myocardial infarction 159
Myocarditis 1, 99
Myoglobinuria 144

Narcotics 60
Nephropathy 121
Neurological manifestations 44, 132
Non-traumatic collapses 23

Overweight 134

Pace maker of heart 14
Papilledema 136
Paroxysmal tachycardia 45
Pathophysiology 20
Peptic ulcer 47
Pesticides 62
Physical performance capacity 83
'Pill' 61
Pilots' death 25
Pneumonencephalogram 44
Pneumonia 86
Pneumothorax 46
Postoperative emboli 78
Pre-coronary care 42
Premature beats 42
Premonitory symptoms 83
Pulmonary edema 122, 130
Pulmonary embolism 88
Purkinje cells 129

Quinine 58
QT interval 108

Race horses 15
Renal failure 58, 123, 138
Respiratory infection 45
Rheumatic fever 67
Rupture of aorta 150
Rupture of heart 19

Sedatives 59
Sickling 48, 134
'Silent' heart disease 25
Sinus arrest 109
Sinus node artery 104
Smoking 63
Spleen infarction 48
Status thymicolymphaticus 157
Steroids 61
Strenuous exercise 84
St. Vitus dance 69
Subarachnoid hemorrhage 46
Subendocardial hemorrhage 127
Subendothelial hemorrhage 43
Sudden death of pilots 25f
Suicide 57
Syncope in pilots 43

Terminal trigger mechanisms 41
Thermoregulation 114, 121, 137

Thiazide diuretics 60
Thrombi 87
Thymus 151
Tonsillitis 45
Toxic hazards 57
Tranquilizers 59
Trauma and rheumatic fever 67
Tuberculosis 45
Tumors 1, 44
T wave 34, 122
Twins 23, 41, 154, 159

Ulcer 47
Unconsciousness 25, 43
Urticaria 45

Valsalva phenomenon 13, 20
Ventricular aneurysm 71
Ventricular automatism 14
Ventricular fibrillation 42

Women pilots 61
Wrestler's death 82

Xanthine oxidase inhibitors 61
Xanthomatosis 41

Authors' Index

Abrahams, A. 16, 24
Abrahams, C. 147
Abernathy, R. S. 147
Agorio, E. 175
Aldersberg, D. 165
Amad, K. 80
Anderson, R. M. 80
Andrews, P. A. 51
Aschoff, L. 158
Austin, M. G. 146
Aylward, R. D. 175

Baetzner, W. 16
Bailey, C. P. 80
Balke, B. 88
Bamford, C. 16
Barber, H. 16, 79
Barlow, J. B. 111
Bartholomew, R. D. 52, 97
Barry, K. G. 147
Barry, M. E. 146
Baumann, H. 16
Baxter, C. R. 147
Bean, W. B. 88
Beck, C. S. 80
Becker, T. 51
Bedford, T. H. B. 174
Beisel, W. R. 147
Benchimol, A. 159
Benedict, R. B. 165
Benson, O. 16, 51
Bergmann, E. 158
Bergmann, G. 16, 24
Bergmeyer, H. U. 146
Bernstein, S. 80

Berry, J. W. 146
Beyer, J. 51, 88
Binder 48
Bing, R. VIII, 4
Blankenhorn, M. A. 146
Blondheim, S. H. 146
Blumgart, H. L. 158
Blumgart, M. 24
Boas, E. P. 16
Bolton, H. E. 80
Bonnett, L. M. 152
Booze, jr. 54
Borst, W, 16
Bosman. C. K. 111
Bougas, J. A. 80
Boulter, E. A. 51
Bourne, G. 88
Brack, E. 16
Brahdy, L. 16
Braunwald, E. 175
Brent, L. B. 175
Bright, E. F. 80
Brown, W. G. 89
Brunner, D. 4
Buchner, F. 88
Burch, G. E. 174
Burger, F. 147
Burger, M. 16, 24
Burton, A. C. 120

Cairns, F. J. 174
Campbell, M. 16
Carter, E. T. 53
Cathcart, R. T. 80
Catherman, R. L. 51

Catlett, G. F. 51
Chapman, D. W. 80
Clark, M. L. 89
Cluver, E. H. 4, 24, 51, 97, 153
Cochrane, J. W. 111
Cohen, L. S. 97
Comeau, W. J. 165
Conley, C. L. 53
Connolly, D. C. VIII
Cooley, D. A. 80
Cooley, J. C. 51
Cooper, K. H. 51
Constantino, J. G. 53
Cowdry, E. V. 157
Cullen, G. E. 146
Currens, H. VIII, 97
Custer, R. P. 146

Dack, S. 17, 66, 88, 89
Davidson, G. M. 16
Davidson, W. H. 51
Davis, A. W. 55
Davis, D. 158
Davis, J. H. 147
De La Place, S. 146
DeMuth, W. E. 80
Denney, M. K. 51
DePasquale, N. P. 174
Derby, I. M. 16
DeSanto, D. A. 88
De Traglia, J. 111
De Vito, J. J. 166
De Wall, R. A. 80
Dietrich, A. 16, 24
Dille, J. R. 51, 57
Dimond, E. G. 159
Dock, W. 66
Doerr, W. 88
Donowho 48
Drake, E. 80, 175
Drazil, V. 88
Duma, R. J. 147
Durnin, J. V. G. A. 120

Edholm, O. G. VIII, 120
Edstroem, G. 70
Effler, D. B. 80
Eldahl, A. 16
Engel, C. E. 51
Enos, W. F. 51, 88
Erikson, E. E. 174
Evans, W. 175

Ferguson, M. 146
Ferris, E. B. 146
Fiebach, R. 16
Field, L. E. 88, 89
Findlay, G. M. 51
Fiorcia, V. 55
Fisher, R. 52, 174
Fisch, C. 111
Fitzgerald, R. P. 89
Fithzhugh, G. 88
Fowler, N. O. 175
Fox, R. H. VIII, 120
Fraimow, W. 80
Frame, B. 111
Fraser, G. R. 111
Freedman, B. L. 89
French, A. J. 66
French, H. 79
Freud, S. F. 52
Froggatt, P. 4, 52, 102
Froment, R. 165
Fuchs 46
Fuenning, S. I. 80
Fuhrman, F. 147
Fulton, W. F. 88
Fulton, Z. M. K. 175
Funkhouser, G. E. 55

Gale, H. 80
Gamstrop, I. 111
Gauss, H. 146
Gazes, P. C. 175
Gentsch, T. O. 80
Gerrard, E. S. 147
Glancy, D. L. 71
Glantz, W. M. 51
Glendy, R. E. 66
Glenn, W. W. L. 80
Giddings, L. W. 80
Giknis, F. L. 159
Gilbert, N. C. 24
Gilman, R. 80
Goedvolk, C. 16
Goldstein, S. 80
Goldys, F. M. 53
Gouze, F. J. 52, 97
Gower 43
Gravenhorst 16
Gray, D. M. 147
Graybiel, A. 52, 88
Green, J. R. 55, 166

Greenstein, J. 52, 64, 80
Grisham, A. 88
Groves, L. K. 80
Gubner, R. 89
Guinet, P. 165
Guthrie, J. 146

Haager, B. 88
Hamilton, B. 88
Hammack, W. J. 147
Hammond, W. H. 120
Han, J. 111
Hardway, R. N. 16
Hart, C. 152
Hartley, P. 16
Hartmann, H. 56
Hawkes, S. Z. 79
Haymaker, W. 146
Heilmann, P. 17
Hellermann, W. 17
Hellerstein, H. K. 52, 80
Helpern, M. 52, 174
Helwig, C. F. 17
Henderson, A. B. 52
Henderson, H. S. 121
Henke, F. 152
Herndon, E. G. 147
Hervey, G. R. VIII, 120
Heyman, C. 17, 24
Higgins, E. A. 55
Hoffman, A. A. 53
Hollman, A. 175
Holmes, R. H. 51, 88
Holt, D. E. 159
Holzmann, M. 17
Hoon, R. S. 89
Horn, H. 88, 89
Howard, J. M. 147
Hueppe, F. 17
Hume, M. 80

Iampietro, P. F. 55

Jaffe, H. L. 17, 66, 89
Jaffe, R. 174
James, T. N. 4, 52, 56, 102, 111, 175
Janelli, D. E. 80
Jarisch 17, 24
Jernigan, J. P. 51
Jervell, A. 175

Joachim, H. 79
Johnson, K. E. 147
Johnson, W. C. 147
Jones 48
Jores, L. 152
Jorgensen, F. 147
Judson, C. F. 175

Kagan, A. 4
Kahler, O. H. 165
Karvonen, M. J. 89
Katz, L. N. 80
Kay, J. H. 80
Kew, M. C. 147
Khanna, P. K. 89
Kidera, G. J. 51
Kihlberg, J. 89
Kimmelstiel, P. 147
King, B. A. 146
Kintzios, J. A. 146
Kirch, E. 17
Kissane, R. W. 80
Klaus, E. J. 17
Klopp, E. 147
Knochel, J. P. 146, 147
Knoll, E. 17
Koerner, M. 54
Kolb, G. 101
Koppisch, E. 174
Korbsch, L. 17
Koskela, A. 89
Krovetz, M. J. 166
Kuller, L. 52, 174

Lachmund, H. 17
Laite, M. B. 174
Lal, M. 89
Lalich, J. 147
Lam, C. R. 80
Lamb, L. E. 52
Lane, J. C. 52
Lange-Nielsen, F. 175
Lauren, E. 174
Laurence, J. 17
Laurie, W. 165
Lehman, W. 165
Lehmus, H. J. 80
Leithead, C. S. 146
Lepel 17
Lev, M. 55, 174
Levin, N. W. 147

Levine, R. J. 80
Levine, S. A. 66
Levy, H. 80
Levy, M. J. 80
Lewis, Th. 17
Lichtlen, P. R. 89
Lilienfeld, A. 52, 174
Liljestrand, G. 17, 24
Lillihei, C. W. 80
Lind, A. R. 146
Lisa, J. R. 17
Livsic, A. M. 4
Longo, E. 80
Lorentz, H. 17
Loughridge, L. W. 147
Lovell, F. W. 53
Lowen, B. 42
Lubarsch, O. 152
Lucke, B. 147
Luke, J. L. 52

McArdle, B. 146
McCurdy, H. J. 17
McFadden, S. 111
McFarland, R. A. 52, 88
McIntosh, D. A. 147
McKenzie, R. T. 17
McKusick, V. A. 165
McPhaul, J. 147
MacDowell, M. 147
MacGibbons, C. B. 51
Mackintosh, R. H. 150
Maegraith, B. G. 146
Malamud, N. 146
Mangiardi, J. L. 80
Manion, W. C. 79
Manning, G. W. 52
Marchard, W. E. 146
Margoliash, E. 146
Marks, H. H. 89
Marsan 55
Marshall, T. K. 4, 52, 102
Martin-Noel 165
Marvin, H. M. 17
Mason, J. K. 52
Master, A. M. 17, 66, 88, 89
Matthes, K. 17
Mattingly, T. W. 79
Mays, A. T. 79
Meessen, H. 89
Mellerowicz, H. 89

Melzer, L. 4, 5, 52, 67, 158
Merrill, J. P. 147
Meyer, K. A. 146
Miller, W. E. 147
Millett, D. 111
Milne, M. D. 147
Moe, G. K. 111
Mohler, S. R. 51–53, 57
Monge, C. C. 52
Monge, C. M. 52
Moore, E. N. 111
Moritz, A. R. 52, 80, 89, 174
Morrow, A. G. 80
Morton, T. C. 146
Muller, E. 17
Mundy, R. L. 147
Munscheck, H. 89
Murch, H. 17

Nelson, M. G. 66
Neptune, W. B. 80
Newman, B. 81
Nichols, H. 80
Nilsen, R. 111
Norman, L. G. 56
Noro, L. 89
Norris, G. W. 175
Nylin, G. 17

O'Brien, J. G. 52
O'Brien, M. M. 146
Oliver, J. 147
Olsen, S. 147
O'Meara, M. P. 147
Orlady, H. 53
Osawa, G. 147
Osborne, R. H. 165
Osler, W. 175
Overholt, B. M. 53

Panico, F. G. 80
Papodopoulos, N. M. 146
Parade, G. W. 24, 158, 165
Pare, J. A. 175
Parmley, L. F. 79
Parsons, Smith, G. 80
Patterson, J. G. 17
Pearce, A. G. E. 146
Pellegrino, E. D. 53
Pende, N. 17
Perkoff, G. T. 147

Peterson, W. L. 51
Petren, T. 24
Phipps, C. 89
Pitts, H. H. 79
Ponsold, A. 4, 17, 97
Post, R. S. 147
Preston, J. B. 111
Pruitt, R. D. 175
Pugh, L. G. C. E. VIII, 53, 112
Purvis, G. S. 79

Rabson, S. M. 174
Randerath, E. 79
Rao, B. D. 89
Rash, J. O. 53
Read, R. C. 51
Reighard, H. L. 53
Reimer, D. 146
Rhoades, E. R. 147
Richards, R. 174
Rigal, R. D. 53
Robb, G. P. 89
Roberts, J. A. F. 165
Roberts, W. C. 71, 80
Robinson, H. W. 146
Robinson, S. VIII
Rokitansky, C. 158
Romeo, J. A. 147
Rook, A. F. 43, 53
Rose, K. D. 80
Ross, G. D. 52, 89, 97
Ross, R. S. 89
Rubberdt, H. 17, 98
Ruberman, W. 42
Rubinstein, A. H. 147
Rush, B. F. 147

Schatz, I. J. 111
Schlesinger, M. J. 158, 165
Schlichter, J. 80
Schlomka, G. 17
Schmidt, A. P. VIII
Schmidt, W. 17, 70
Schoneberg, H. 17
Schreuder, O. B. 53
Schrier, R. W. 121
Schurmann 17
Schwiegk, S. 24
Scully, N. M. 80
Seftel, M. C. 147
Seiling, V. 147

Seipel, J. H. 53
Shackman, R. 147
Shafrir, E. 146
Shanklin, D. R. 166, 174
Shaw, L. D. 97, 56
Sheldon, S. 174
Shipley, J. 24
Shipley, R. 24
Shulack, N. R. 17
Siegel, M. B. 53, 54, 57
Siegel, P. V. 53
Simonson, E. 89
Singh, I. 89
Singh, M. D. 159
Sjostrand, S. 24
Skjoldborg, H. 147
Smith, E. W. 53
Smith, L. H. 147
Sobel, S. 147
Spain, D. M. 89
Spicer, F. W. 17
Spilsbury, B. 4, 17, 24, 98
Stapleton, J. F. 89
Stefan, H. 17
Stembridge, V. A. 51
Stephenson, G. E. 18
Sternby, N. 4
Stone, F. 80
Study, R. S. 175
Sullivan, B. H. 53
Sullivan, J. J. 80
Sundquist, A. B. 80
Surawicz, B. 53
Suzman, M. M. 24
Swann, R. C. 147

Tannen, R. L. 121
Tanner, J. M. 120
Taylor, W. J. 166
Telling, M. 80
Templeton, J. W. 80
Teschan, P. E. 147
Thornell, H. E. 52
Tisher, C. C. 121
Titus, J. L. VIII
Tolentino, P. 80
Toole, A. L. 80
Torkelson, L. 55
Townsend, F. M. 51, 53
Tracey, A. 147
Traum, A. H. 89
Trigg, J. W. 147

Turell, D. J. 52

Umberger, E. L. 52

Vaughan, J. A. 55
Veregge, J. E. 52
Vertel, R. M. 146
Vignon, G. 165
Vihert, A. M. 4
Visscher, M. B. 24

Wallgren, A. 175
Ward, O. C. 111, 175
Warburg, E. 79
Warden, H. E. 80
Wasastjerma, E. 152
Weber, A. 88
Weber, R. 165
Webster, J. G. 53
Wedgwood, J. 88
Welsh, P. P. 89
Wendkos, M. H. 175
Wentz, A. E. 53, 63
Werkmeister, R. 18
Wern, J. T. 24
Wescott, R. N. 80
Westling, H. 111

Weyrich, G. 174
White, D. VIII
White, P. D. 18, 66, 97, 165
Whitehouse, R. H. 120
Whiteman, H. W. 159
Willcox, W. H. 146
Willett 57
Williams, D. J. 43, 53, 80
Williams, L. N. 53
Williams, W. C. 52, 97
Wilde, A. 18
Winblad, S. 175
Wise, N. B. 165
Wolf, P. L. VIII, 4
Wolf, W. 157
Wolff, H. S. VIII, 120
Woods, J. D. 165
Wooler, G. H. 80
Wooten, I. D. P. 147

Yarnell 71
Yater, W. M. 89
Young, D. 149

Zamcheck, N. 52, 89, 174
Zivin 55
Zinsser, H. F. 80
Zoll, P. M. 89